SOBRIETY IN BLACK

CONFESSIONS OF A RETIRED ALCOHOLIC

HANIEF SATERFIELD

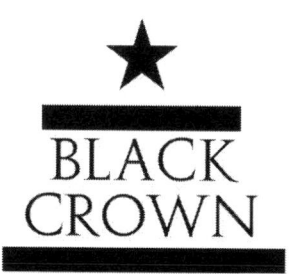

Copyright © 2022, All Rights Reserved

Black Crown Publishing
Desoto, TX 75115
1-214-702-6383
www.sobrietyinblack.com
©2022 by Black Crown Publishing
All rights reserved

Printed in the United States of America

Duplicating this publication is illegal, except for the assessment tools and questionnaires that appear in the appendixes. Please do not copy any other material without written permission from the publisher.

ISBN 978-0-9987975-2-6 (Paperback)
ISBN 978-0-9987975-3-3 (Ebook)

Cover design by H2 Media Services
Interior design by H2 Media Services

Be Sober, Be Vigilant

*Be sober, be vigilant;
because your adversary the devil,
as a roaring lion, walketh about,
seeking whom he may devour:*

*Whom resist steadfast in the faith,
knowing that the same afflictions
are accomplished in your brethren that
are in the world.* - 1 Peter 5:8-9

*Blessed be the LORD my strength,
which teacheth my hands to war,
and my fingers to fight* - Psalms 144:1

*For we wrestle not against flesh and blood,
but against principalities, against powers,
against the rulers of the darkness of this world,
against spiritual wickedness in high places.* - Ephesians 6:12

*Therefore let us not sleep, as do others;
but let us watch and be sober.* - 1 Thessalonians 5:6

This book is dedicated to my children:
Hanief II, Serenity, and Jihad

Contents

Introduction 7
The History of Alcohol in Black American Society 11
   Alcohol as a Weapon of Oppression 18
   Alcohol and the African Slave Trade 20
Blacks and Booze in the Present Day 23
Tales From the Bottom of the Bottle 25
   My First Sip: Thanksgiving, 1985 25
   Me vs. The Mountain 32
Step 1: BEGIN 44
   What is your LOCALE? (Level Of Change and Life Environment) .. 45
      Level 1: Pre-Contemplation: 47
      Level 2: Contemplation: 50
      Level 3: Preparation and Determination: 52
      Level 4: Action 54
      Level 5: Maintenance 56
   Relapse: What to consider 57
The 12 Superpowers of Sobriety 64
What Brings You to the Bottle? 75
Step 2: LEARN 86
   The Addiction: 87
The Drinker's Loop 92
The Drinker's Jacket: 95
Changing your Social Identity 95
   The 'Drunk Jacket': How your alcoholism becomes your identity 97
   Sobriety Reaction Types 101
Discovering your "Why?" 109
   The Crutch and the Cheerleader 109

Convertible Crush: Kela's Story 111
Why do you want to stop drinking? 114
Alcohol Ugly: The symptoms 118
Step 3: ACT 121
    Handling H.A.T.E. (High Addiction Triggering Elements) 124
    Addiction Triggers 125
    Emotional Triggers 125
    Situational Triggers 128
    Environmental Triggers 132
Step 4: CONNECT 138
    That which is monitored is managed 139
    Building Your Village 147
        Sobriety as a team sport 147
        Your Sober Social Support Group 158
Step 5: KEEP 167
    The Relapses 168
    Sobriety is Never Owned 169
    Renew, Review, Refocus and Reclaim 173
List of activities 181
    Types of Hobbies 183
    Your Hobbies 183
    Medicinal Options 185
    According to the CDC: 187
Recovering Loudly 190
Appendix 197

Introduction

In 1996, I celebrated my 21st birthday (AKA my transition into "Adulthood") with some E&J and Coke and never looked back. It wasn't until about two months before my mother died in 2003 that I found out alcoholism ran through her and my father's side of the family. My addiction then made sense because whenever I found a new passion and I fell hard. Usually, any newfound passion I found would dissipate after a certain time, but alcohol stuck and grew into an addiction. It wasn't until I caught three DUIs (one case I beat), made multiple failed attempts at sobriety, and witnessed the degeneration of my life that I found the strength to begin my current sobriety streak on July 24, 2011. I am proud to say I have lived an alcohol-free life ever since.

During my first attempt at sobriety, I told everyone that I had quit drinking. I wanted to express my commitment to everyone, so they knew I was serious and did not offer me any liquor or beer. My friends and family lauded my effort but were skeptical, given my propensity to swim in the bottle. During my first attempt to stop drinking, friends often treated me like a pastor at the party when drinking in my presence. My fraternity brothers and close friends agreed to support me by not offering me drinks, and my wife seemed to support my decision at the time. Although I initially thought everyone was in full support of my decision, I noticed things that at the time felt odd but would later reveal dynamics I had not considered when I began my journey to sobriety.

It was apparent that my old drinking buddies began to feel uneasy around me. They stopped joking when I used to get drunk with them. I began to feel like an outsider whose presence was no longer welcome but tolerated. They treated me like a different person, not like the Hanif they knew and loved or the identity I had crafted for myself inside my alcoholism. I began questioning my intrinsic value, which affected how I saw myself and felt about my need to drink. I became tempted to drink to regain the comradeship I previously had with my friends. My first attempt at sobriety lasted a couple of months, but after prolonged cravings and feelings of alienation, I soon returned to the bottle. I didn't stay there, however.

Now that I have been sober for over a decade, many people have asked me how I did it. Those who knew the old me are now convinced that my perpetual sobriety is absolute. And now, some wish to obtain it for themselves. I have realized the value in not only sharing my story to help others but also in taking a comprehensive look at the dynamics of my relationship with alcohol and the dynamics within it that are unique to Black society. I have come to realize that in America, Black people have a unique set of circumstances and obstacles we must overcome when it comes to alcohol that other groups do not have. These differences come from the history Black people share with the country itself, predicated on predatory racism, socialization, and the abusive relationship between Black people, alcohol, and American society.

This is a book about my not-so illustrious career as an alcoholic, my failed attempts at sobriety, and the mindset that made my retirement in recovery sustainable. There are many books on how to attain sobriety. Still, not many expose and address the historical and inevitable factors that come with not only being an alcoholic but also being a Black alcoholic. Just as being a Black mother or Black father in America can be the most challenging title due to the burdens of racial socialization, seeking sobriety as a Black alcoholic has unique challenges unknown to any other group of people. I will use the following pages to evaluate cultural and societal factors as they relate to the consumption of alcohol among Black Americans. These individual factors, and others, will be discussed further in the book as an offering to anyone that has tirelessly worked to earn a life of sobriety.

The History of Alcohol in Black American Society

One of my earliest memories of television commercials growing up was seeing Billy Dee Williams charismatically promote Colt 45 Malt Liquor. At 11 years of age, I had no real idea about liquor or any desire to drink beer; I just knew that the ladies loved them some Billy Dee Williams. The commercials were scripted to attribute his fascinating life, favorable looks, and fortune with the ladies to drinking this beer. In one commercial, Billy Dee stated, "There are two rules to remember when trying to have a good time: Rule #1 never run out of Colt 45. Rule #2, never forget rule #1."

In the next scene, Billy is holding a can of Colt while asking, "You want to know why you should keep Colt 45 on hand?" (Female hand enters camera shot to grab Colt can from Billy Dee) "You never know when friends might show up." Cut to a fine, light-skinned female resembling Whitley from *A Different World* smiling while holding what used to be Billy Dee's Colt. He then stated, "I don't claim you can have a better time with Colt 45 than without it," as Whitley looks seductively at Billy Dee, then at the viewer through the screen. "...but why take chances?" he responds. Then Billy Dee says, "Never mind that I'm a world-famous actor, good-looking, and filthy rich. Fact is, I *need* Colt 45 to be me, and you need it to become me!"

The crazy thing is that he was telling the truth about what he was paid by Colt, the TV time, and personal accouterments afforded through his work and association with Colt 45. Today, many professional athletes, musicians, and other entertainers make more money through endorsements than through their professional work. During shows with high African American viewership, Black male celebrities have been used to endorse and promote alcohol products in ads. According to a 2010 study on youth exposure to alcohol advertising in national magazines, "Youths' exposure to distilled spirits advertising was approximately equal to that of adults. African-American youths were exposed to 32% more alcohol advertising in magazines than youths in general, although they had slightly less exposure than African-American adults." At that time, most men in Black society would have loved to be Billy Dee, and all the ladies in our family would have loved to be with Billy Dee—and the advertisers knew it.

In the mid-70s and 80s, many Black celebrities were paid to promote Schlitz Malt Liquor Bull to Black Americans. Below is a list of the entertainers that were constantly paraded in front of the screen during regularly scheduled TV programs to promote "The Bull":

Rufus Thomas

The Commodores

Kool & the Gang

The Platters

Teddy Pendergrass

Richard Roundtree

Antonio Fargas

The Drifters

Skyy

The Four Tops

Gregory Hines

The Spinners

Wilson Pickett

While the few all-white Schlitz commercials I did find promoted consumption as a one-off for a unique experience. For instance, two of the commercials involved a prisoner being offered a last request before death where, of course, they chose to sip "The Bull." Conversely, most of the Schlitz commercials targeting Black audiences did not portray drinking as a special event but as an everyday occurrence—promoting drinking to the Black community as **a way of life**. This advertising method helped further the idea of regular drinking in the Black community. Although we drink less than other ethnicities, there was a clear imbalance in the amount of advertising dedicated to the Black community. We had a naturally lower tolerance for alcohol, but we were socially encouraged to drink more. We also suffer more tragedies because of our alcohol consumption, from disproportionate DUI arrests and convictions to increased gun violence.

In the 90s, Hip-Hop took over the mainstream music landscape as an unstoppable force in the entertainment industry. Every top-ten-selling rap artist or group was getting paid well to endorse beer and liquor in all forms. On team malt liquor, you had the beloved St. Ides with commercials from the Notorious B.I.G. to Wutang Clan, Snoop Dogg, Warren G, and Nate Dogg. Eazy E had the '8 Ball Rollin,' and DJ Quik was off that Tanqueray. In the mixed drink sector, Tupac was pushing "Thug Passion," French connections, and Incredible Hulks, and they were being requested in every club in Southern California. To get the conscious sector in on it, Budweiser held the Budweiser Superfest and made a poster series called 'Kings and Queens of Africa' that hung in many Black homes. These posters were beautifully artistic renditions of our African ancestors, such as Mansa Musa, Hannibal, and King Tut, with a paragraph on their attributes and accomplishments. If you were born between 1965 and 1980, you probably smile while going down memory lane reading this paragraph. Everything I have mentioned in the previous sections has two things in common: They are inextricably tied to Black culture and are all related to the sale and marketing of alcohol.

In 1992, the year I graduated high school, the Los Angeles Times ran an article on the shrewd marketing and sales of malt liquor in "ethnic neighborhoods." At the time, debates were going on over the targeted advertising of the cheap malt liquor known to be more potent than regular beer. It seemed apparent that the more potent brew was being marketed in Black and Latino communities without consequence. According to a study by Shanken Communications Inc. of New York City, Blacks made up 10% of beer drinkers but were 28% of the malt liquor consumers.

Below is a list of popular beer and malt liquor brands and their alcohol content.

ALCOHOL CONTENT OF POPULAR BRANDS
(in percent)

Beers	Malt Liquors
Coors: 4.5　　Miller: 4.6　　Budweiser: 4.7	King Cobra: 6.0　　Schlitz Red Bull: 6.9　　St. Ides: 8.0

Source: Center for Science in the Public Interest; Jobson Publishing Corp.

Can you name any white brand ambassadors for liquor companies besides NASCAR drivers? I believe that America has been on a longstanding campaign to promote intoxicants to Black people disproportionately. If you ask a white person born in the same era to name a concert series or significant annual event with a primarily white audience named after a liquor company or an alcoholic beverage company, they may draw a blank. For white people, alcohol consumption is promoted as a rare thing to be indulged in during special events such as celebrations and sporting events. I have often seen alcohol consumption promoted as a way of life for the Black community. Although studies have shown that we are more genetically sensitive to alcohol (we get intoxicated faster with less alcohol when compared to other ethnic groups) and beer has been marketed to us rigorously over the broad course of American history.

Alcohol as a Weapon of Oppression

I remember learning about two techniques in history class that the Pilgrims used to take over Native American land and subjugate the Native population. One technique was the handing out blankets laced with smallpox—one of the earliest acts of germ warfare—and the second was the introduction of hard liquor to the tribesmen. European colonizers knew that to take over Native land, they had to weaken the mental resolve of their prey. Offering alcohol to the tribal chiefs in the name of "goodwill" and "celebration," the Europeans were able to affect the state of mind of Indians, who were then unable to protect their land effectively. Although Native Americans drank wine, the high grain alcohol introduced to them by the pilgrims was ten times stronger than what they were used to.

According to Dr. Fred Beuvais in his article "American Indians and Alcohol," before European colonization, Native Americans were naive to the effects of grain alcohol as they only produced less potent beers and other fermented beverages for ceremonial purposes. When the European colonizers showed up, they capitalized on this naiveté by producing and encouraging the consumption of distilled spirits and wine with potent levels of alcohol. Their tactic was to provide free alcohol during trading sessions (the conducting of business) to garner an advantage in negotiations. They also made it a medium of trade, often using it in exchange for highly coveted animal skins and other resources. In the beginning, White colonists would overdrink with the Native Americans to model the social overconsumption they wanted to see among their prey. As with the Africans, Europeans encouraged using their foreign alcohol because they already knew of its debilitating effect. When these groups understood the tactic, a pattern of overdrinking had already been established.

Alcohol and the African Slave Trade

"*Owners of slavers carried enslaved people to South Carolina and brought home naval stores for their shipbuilding, or to the West Indies and brought home molasses or other colonies and hogsheads. The molasses was made into the highly prized New England rum and shipped in these hogsheads to Africa for more enslaved people*" – W.E.B. Dubois

Although American slavery is historically associated with Southern states, Northern states also had a role in trading enslaved Africans. In his book, *The Suppression of the Slave Trade*, W.E.B. Dubois discusses New England states and their involvement in the rum-slave trade. New England was known throughout America for its premium rum. While the use of enslaved people was discouraged in the North, that didn't stop New England states such as Rhode Island and Massachusetts from being involved in the trade and transportation of enslaved Africans through the use of rum as a currency of trade and its manufacture, and the bribery of slave trading tribes in Africa.

My Uncle, James Bliese, once told me about how during apartheid in South Africa, beer was readily available to the oppressed Black masses. Instead of public water fountains, spigots strategically placed in the settlements by South African invading forces dispensed alcoholized water to keep the Black Africans inebriated. All the captives, including the children, had little to no access to pure water and were therefore left to depend on the readily available "beer water" for survival.

Below is a list of legal acts that directly spoke about the rum-slave trade in New England:

1704, October. Maryland: 20s. Duty Act

"An Act imposing Three Pence per Gallon on Rum and Wine, Brandy and Spirits; and Twenty Shillings per Poll for Negroes; for raising a Supply to defray the Public Charge of this Province;

and Twenty Shillings per Poll on Irish Servants, to prevent the importing too great several Irish Papists into this Province." Revived in 1708 and 1712. Bacon, Laws, 1704, ch. xxxiii.

1708, Ch. xvi.; 1712, Ch. xxii.

1710, Dec. 28. Pennsylvania: 40s. Duty Act

"*An impost Act, laying a duty on Negroes, wine, rum, and other spirits, cyder, and vessels.*" *Repealed by order in Council Feb. 20, 1713. Carey and Bioren, Laws, I. 82; Bettle, Notices of Negro Slavery, in Penn. Hist. Soc. Mem. (1864), I. 415.*

Pennsylvania: Prohibitive Duty Act. 1712, June 7

"*A supplementary Act to an act, entitled, An Impost Act, laying a duty on Negroes, rum,*" *etc. Disallowed by Great Britain, 1713. Carey and Bioren, Laws, I. 87, 88. Cf. Colonial Records (1852), II. 553.*

Blacks and Booze in the Present Day

The campaign to keep Black America intoxicated evolved. In the early 2000s the use of liquid codeine, promethazine, and Sprite, marketed as a new product called "Lean," was promoted in rap music as a viable alternative to alcohol. Similar to alcohol, the physiological effects of lean include mild "euphoric side effects", along with "motor-skill impairment, lethargy, drowsiness, and a dissociative feeling from all other parts of the body."

In an article by Kaiser Health News entitled, "Opioids Like 'Lean' Permeate Hip-Hop Culture, but Dangers Are Downplayed," writer Chaseedaw Giles cited a 2020 sage journal research paper that found a significant increase in prescription opioid overdose deaths among Black people. This paper also noted that the death rate almost tripled between 1999 and 2017.

Lean comes in a wide range of colors reminiscent of Kool-Aid. I believe that album covers and songs promoting *Lean* written by kids not old enough to drive helped to cultivate a crop of new young addicts consuming a substance that is as potent and damaging as alcohol. Conversely, pharmaceutical companies benefit from this new industry as the creators of both the sickness and the cure. I'm sure Black teens don't have a network of laboratories where they bind chemicals together to manufacture Promethazine. At best, these kids are purchasing from a wholesaler/distributor that is getting it at a bulk premium rate from the manufacturer cooking it up in some laboratory. I have always found it interesting that the media reports on these drug scourges, and the prosecution primarily focuses their attention on the street level dealers and addicts while paying no time and attention to the manufacturers responsible for the product's origination. Unfortunately, as long as money is made from addiction, there will always be an industry ready to profit from the damage. My guess is the target market for lean looks nothing like the children of those responsible for the manufacture and distribution of codeine and promethazine

Tales From the Bottom of the Bottle

My First Sip: Thanksgiving, 1985

At age ten, I vividly remember my Uncle Hank sneaking me a sip of beer. One Thanksgiving holiday, he was in the kitchen drunk and jovial as usual, bugging my mom while she was cooking. Suddenly, my uncle decided to slip me a lil' taste of his Budweiser. I always remembered seeing cans of Coors and Budweiser floating throughout the house during holidays and adult party nights my parents would host. Admittedly, I may have asked for a sip from my uncle, knowing he would oblige since my father would have killed me for asking. As a middle child growing up in the 80s, my job was to be the rebellious knucklehead among the siblings. I was the first to break curfew, break both my arms doing shit I had no business doing, get caught stealing, almost burn down a field, and smoke cigarettes.

The beer tasted nasty, but I felt like a grown up for a moment as I raised the can to my lips. After a couple of sips, my mother slapped the can of beer out of my hand and preceded to yell at my uncle adamantly yet playfully for "hooking me up." My mom fake argued with my uncle before laughing it off as I was exiled out of the kitchen. I quickly shifted my focus to running around the house, looking for other trouble to get into.

Riding Dirty Looking for Birdy: Wet and Reckless

I received my first DUI charge in 2003 in the parking lot of a club. I was by myself in my 1982 Cutlass Supreme when, after a day of drinking, I decided to go to Godfathers, a local nightclub where a friend of mine, The Dirdy Birdy, was set to perform. I was driving (swerving) down a street in Ontario, looking for the club, around 11:30. I had passed the club multiple times before realizing where it was located. As I pulled into the parking lot, I noticed a cop car following me. As I started pulling into a parking spot in front of the club, the police hit their lights. Admittedly, I had been swerving, slowing and making multiple U turns while looking for the club, so the cops knew I wasn't merely lost, but lost and loaded. While trying to blame my suspiciously erratic driving on being lost, my breath snitched on me as it screamed from the mountaintops like Samuel Jackson, "This motherfucker is drunk as hell!" I could hear Dirdy Birdy in the background performing on stage inside as I was administered a Breathalyzer test, subsequently arrested, and placed in the cop car to be sent to the local drunk tank. I attempted to fight the DUI charge since I was parked when I was stopped, and, according to the breathalyzer, my alcohol level barely exceeded the legal limit. With this, I was able to get the charge reduced to a "Wet and Reckless." In California, a Wet and Reckless is a lesser charge with a fine that is not reflected on your record with a condition that I not re-offend in the next seven years. If I did reoffend in that time my original charge would be bumped up to a DUI, and I would end up with two DUIs. I would re-offend in subsequent years.

The Takeaway: Red Flags Matter

Take notice of the red flags that pop up in your life. Red flags are warning signs that may point to a destructive pattern of behavior. By the time I had my first arrest, I had plenty of nights where I had got too drunk, lost things, and crashed vehicles without getting caught. This was the first time an outside entity had caught me in the act of drinking and driving. Had I recognized the red flag in this scenario, I could have started to make the necessary changes to avoid the pain I would endure due to abusing alcohol in the future. The worst thing that can happen for an alcoholic, or anyone engaging in destructive behavior, is getting away with it because every time you do, it reinforces the chances of you doing it repeatedly. We continue to take risks until our number is called and we are finally caught, or suffer a more significant consequence.

If you are thinking about quitting alcohol, think about all that you have gotten away with while drunk and what your life would look like if you hadn't gotten away. What are the potential worst-case scenarios of your past actions? Could you have died, killed someone, or been locked up due to risks you have taken with alcohol in the past? Whom would it affect in your life? What negative consequences would you avoid entirely with a dash of sobriety? These are the questions you want to ask yourself and red flags offer you an opportunity to do so.

Cleopatra's

In 2003, my brother from another mother, Steve opened a women's clothing store named after his first-born daughter, *Sasha's Boutique*. I had always aspired to be an entrepreneur and was inspired by Steve's business acumen.

Sasha's sat on the corner of Riverside and Baseline in the city of Rialto. It was located in a supermarket shopping center, two doors down from a Jamaican restaurant and three doors down from a liquor store, so you already knew what was going on...daily. It was *the hotspot* back then. Business would be going on in the front and staff, local customers, and friends from the area would hang out in the front parking lot drinkin', chillin' and talkin' shit. Steve was always about his business so he'd be making sure employees were good and the money was getting made, while popping out to contribute to the shit talking of course.

Two years after opening, Steve offered me the opportunity to go into business with him, selling women's accessories at the shop. He sold the clothing and shoes while I supplied and sold the hats, purses, sunglasses, and belts. Soon after, I started selling Nextel phones affectionately known as "chirps" because these phones had a walkie-talkie function that would chirp during use. Ask any Generation Xer about Nextel chirps, and they'll probably light up as they reminisce about these beautiful machines. Due to the way I was pushing the Nextels I became known as "The Chirpman." I always wore a sweater with my chirp number on the front, advertising it freely like Houston rapper Mike Jones' who promoted his phone number in many of his songs.

About a year after I entered the shop, another good brother we affectionately called "Rasta" rented space in *Sasha's* where he sold mixtapes and throwback jerseys. As the store became a fixture in the neighborhood, Steve, decided to lease out another spot three doors down and open a soul food restaurant and lounge called *Cleopatra's Diner*. He acquired a liquor license to sell beer and wine for the diner, which meant we would stay drinking. At *Cleopatra's*, local folk and visitors enjoyed eating, drinking, and socializing. Sometimes a band would come through and play live music. He also held a few fraternity parties and Ladies' Nights there.

I spent many days selling items out of *Sasha's* to locals in the community and then going to *Cleopatra's* to drink, eat and socialize with customers and locals that would stop by to hang out. Among the list of locals that would frequent the spot (primarily on weekends) was a local baller that would come in and buy pitchers of beer for everybody in the building when he showed up. I honestly can't remember his name, as I was often drunk when I saw him, so we'll call him James. James was a cool guy with a sense of humor, a positive vibe, a generous spirit and a constant appetite for alcohol so he would keep the drinks flowing.

During one long Friday night of drinking at Cleopatra's, James had been focusing on one particular woman. She came with a friend that ended up leaving her stranded. James offered to give her a ride home but was visibly intoxicated. She rejected the offer, taking note of James drunkenness to which he replied "I may be drunk, but I always make it where I need to go because I drive better when I'm drunk. (You read that right, *better)*. We all laughed, but she still refused. He ended up leaving saying he was going to stop by another place on the way home. That was the last time we saw James alive.

The next day, the newspaper reported that James had run into a telephone pole at freeway speed after leaving a club only a few blocks from *Cleopatra's*. The impact severed his car and body in half. Had that woman taken him up on his offer, she would have died alongside him. This was a sobering event. James was a good brother with a drinking problem and for it he paid the ultimate price.

Me vs. The Mountain

To get to my girlfriend's house, I had to drive through Reche Canyon. Reche Canyon was a five-mile stretch of road between two mountains that connected two major cities: Moreno Valley and San Bernardino. I went to this canyon daily in my 1993 blue Mazda 323 Hatchback, usually drunk and late at night after work when I was ready to see my girlfriend at the time. To exit the canyon, I had to drive up a winding two-way road around a mountain that would spit me out into the city of Moreno Valley on the other side.

I spent the night at my girl's house and woke up to the sound of her yelling for me from downstairs. "Hanief!" Hungover, I begrudgingly got out of bed and went downstairs to ask her why she was yelling. She asked, "What happened last night...." Looking at her confused, she said, "...to your car Hanief. What happened?" I looked out the door and saw nothing wrong with the car.

From the house I could only see one side of my car. After shooting my girl a perplexed look of irritated confusion, she told me to inspect the other side. As I slowly walked out to give my car a 360, an increasing feeling of terror bubbled up in my stomach. Then, my girlfriend said, "By the way, your mom called and said that the police have your wallet and a few of your belongings. You need to go to the station to get your things."

Upon further inspection, I realized that the other side of the car facing the street was FUBAR (F*cked Up Beyond All Repair). The driver's side door could not open, and the window was busted. Before seeing this, I had no recollection of anything happening the night before, but once I stared at my damaged car, bits and pieces of the night started returning to me.

Then it all hit me...

As I circled the mountain on my way out of the canyon, I momentarily blacked out, crossed the ongoing lane, and sideswiped the mountain. Luckily, no oncoming traffic was turning that corner, sparing my life. My car was no match for the mountain. The driver-side door was crushed into the frame of the car exploding the window. The blown tire woke me out of my drunken stupor. After being jolted awake, I remember pulling over and stopping in horror. I quickly realized I couldn't open the door to check my tire, so I jumped out through the hole where my car window used to reside.

I looked around and luckily found no witnesses or approaching vehicles, as it was around

3 a.m. Fearing a cop might pull up and find me drunk next to my wrecked yet still a functional car, I flew into action to replace the tire and get out of there! I could not afford another DUI as this was the second time I ran into an inanimate object: first, the center median, and now a mountain? Not good.

The spare tire was in the trunk under the floor, but as drunks usually become hoarders over time, my trunk was full of random junk as well as my video camera, overnight bag, an illegal double-edged punch dagger, and clothes. I frantically threw everything in my trunk onto the street without a second thought because I needed to get out of there fast before being discovered! After replacing the blown tire, I threw the flat tire into the now empty trunk, jumped back through the window like a NASCAR driver and sped away from the scene.

As I stood in my in front of my wrecked car my I began to wonder how the police were able to locate my mother. The police informed her that my wallet had been found in the middle of the road earlier that morning. In proper drunken form, I somehow left my wallet in the street with the contents of my trunk, which I failed to put back in the car. The police left instructions for me to go to the police station to retrieve my things, which I did while sober. *Side note to some: Although I did receive my ID, the money in my wallet, my video camera, and double edge knife were all missing.*

It became evident that, like my car, there were things in my life that were damaged and needed repair. When intoxicated, you often fail to notice how bad you look. Usually, this is because either folks won't say anything for fear of you getting angry, you do things that irritate people, or you're hanging around other people who share the same problems. Therefore, being honest with yourself about how your addiction affects those around you is important. Talk to people who will be honest with you and surround yourself with people who have similar experiences so that they may shed light on aspects of your addiction that you may not see.

A friend of mine once told me about how after a night out, his date told him the next day that she liked him but was turned off by his intoxicated state. Because he saw her as a higher caliber woman than he was used to dating, he realized that if he wanted to raise the standard of all things around him, it was better for him to pursue sobriety. His tastes and quality of life have improved since he chose to live alcohol-free. He now notices just how bad intoxication looks when he goes out to events with a sober mind, seeing others intoxicated.

So many simple tweaks of fate could have left me dead, paralyzed, or incarcerated for the rest of my life. I was fortunate to only be out $200 cash and a video camera. I could have ended up like Olivia Culbreath, who got drunk and killed six people, including her sister, when she drove the wrong way down a freeway. Olivia was 21 at the time and just got her license back after a five-year suspension due to a DUI she received at age 16.

- Imagine waking up in the hospital to find out you killed six people the night before and getting sentenced to 30 years to life in prison?

- Imagine being sentenced to 50 years in prison like Amber Perera, who was driving drunk on the Selmon Expressway and slammed into the Felipek family. The crash killed Luiz, Rita, and their eight-year-old daughter Giorgia Felipek.
- Imagine being Mathew Carrier, who, after a documented history of drunk driving arrests, killed five in Livingston County, Michigan, in May of 2017. According to the coroner, the passenger, Tina Tinto, burned to death in her car. Mathew was sentenced to 55 years in prison.
- Or former Los Vegas Raiders Receiver Henry Ruggs III who could face 50 years in prison after rear-ending another car at 156 mph, killing 23 year old Tina Tintor who burned to death while trapped inside her wrecked vehicle.

If you have ever been arrested for driving under the influence chances are you have driven drunk many more times. According to the FBI, a drunk driver will drive 80 times under the influence before their first arrest. Any of the above scenarios could have very quickly become my story. It took a lot of self-reflection to understand the gravity of the risks I took with my life and those of others. It is the reason I have decided to speak about my own experiences.

Center Median Mash Up

On one occasion, I woke up in the middle of the night craving a drink and something to eat. Although I was already drunk, I decided to search for more liquor. Two minutes after getting onto the freeway, I almost rear-ended a car that stopped abruptly in front of me. Trying to avoid the car, I swerved left and hit the center median, knocking my car out of commission. Although I was physically okay, I knew I was intoxicated and that it was just a matter of time before the police would show up.

When the police arrived and asked what happened, I attempted to tell them that a car had sideswiped me. I explained that the vehicle sped off and that they should go pursue the suspects. I was "acting" frantically hoping they would quickly speed off to track down the supposed assailant. Needless to say, that bullshit did not work. I was tested, failed, handcuffed, and once again sent to the drunk tank.

While being processed, I ran into someone I went to high school working at the jail who looked at my name and said, "Hanief?" It's been forever. How are you?" I looked at her with embarrassed frustration as if to say, "How the fuck does it look like I'm doing?" But the words I really said were, "Hey" Isn't this lovely? LOL!" "Don't feel bad," she said. "You'd be surprised how many classmates and teachers I've seen come through here, some for much worse than a DUI."

This DUI arrest resulted in my first wet and reckless case being upgraded to a DUI, which resulted in an automatic 18-month suspension of my driver's license and a mandated alcohol treatment program. My wife had to drive me to my mandatory court-appointed AA meetings one day a week for 18 months. That was, of course, a low time in my life but a time that was needed to slow me down. Although I tried to quit drinking I soon relapsed.

The Takeaway

As I sank further into my career as an alcoholic, I began to increase the number of bad habits in my life. I began to become dishonest to avoid dealing with my problem. I lied to an officer to avoid arrest and then to my wife to take attention away from my alcoholism. I became increasingly irritable when I didn't have alcohol, so I resorted to smoking cigarettes and Black and Mild's occasionally, even knowing that my mother had died of lung cancer. A suspended driver's license meant depending on others for transportation, as this all happened before the advent of Uber and Lyft. This meant that I made others, including my wife, relatives, and friends, share in the burden of the consequences of my actions.

The court mandated 18-month alcohol treatment program was conducive to putting me on a better track the second time. The program gave me a perspective about alcoholism and alcoholics that I did not have before. One thing that surprised me was the number of "everyday" people I saw in the meetings.

When I was dropped off at the first meeting, I expected to see a bunch of dirty, physically run-down drunks, drug addicts, and homeless people in the group. I had a stereotype in my head about what alcoholics looked like that was wholly dispelled when I walked into the meeting room.

I remember seeing a nice BMW in the parking lot along with other nice cars. I sat next to a guy I thought to be the instructor as he had a suit on and was clean-cut. Come to find out, he was a fellow offender who was a local attorney. I also met college students, homemakers, and soccer moms mandated to meetings because of multiple DUI convictions, just like me. In all honesty, I was amazed at how normal these people looked! I almost felt ashamed of my preconceived notions but had come to realize that the disease we call alcoholism does not discriminate. It is no respecter of gender, race, creed, color, or socioeconomic status. Anyone can fall victim.

I am proud to say that I have been alcohol-free since July 24th, 2011! I attempted to stop drinking alcohol and relapsed three times before officially kicking my drinking habit. It wasn't until I received a third DUI that would potentially land me in jail that I took inventory of my relapses to uncover the reason for my failure to stay sober. After beating the third case, and by the grace of God, I decided that my children would never know me to be a drinker. I made my final attempt at sobriety by first examining my past failures to figure out what I was going to do differently so that I could retire from the life of an alcoholic. Aside from my children, sobriety is the greatest gift God has ever given me.

The purpose of this book is to share my story and arm the reader with tools for establishing and sustaining a life of sobriety. The sobriety mindset is a transition to a permanent way of living. To maintain sobriety, one must have a correct understanding of everything and everyone that is affected by their addiction *and* their sobriety. It is more than just tactics and techniques but understanding and preparation. Just like retiring from a job you have wrapped your life around, the time and feelings attached to your addiction must be addressed to gain the one thing needed for a sober life: control. Once the transition is complete, it becomes easier to maintain because, like addiction, it becomes a part of you. The first step in living a sober life is important as none of the other steps can occur without the first. You must determine and accept that you have a problem before being able to fix it. Once this happened to me, I began to take the road I will be outlining in the following pages: the road toward…

– Sobriety In Black –

Begin

Learn

Act

Connect

Keep

Step 1: BEGIN

I got my start by giving myself a start.
~Madame C.J. Walker

What is your LOCALE?

(Level Of Change and Life Environment)

lo·cale /lo·kal/ noun

A place where something happens or is set or has associated events.

For any GPS-based app (like Google Maps) to give you directions to a preferred destination, there are two pieces of information it needs: your current location and your chosen destination. Without either piece of information, the app cannot give you adequate directions. A journey to sobriety operates in the same way. You must know your location to craft a plan with the best chance of success. Have you accepted that you have a drinking problem, or are you not sure? Are you ready and willing to make the changes necessary to live a life of sobriety? Also, do the people you hang around or associate with contribute to your drinking? Will they support your path to sobriety? What triggers in your life cause you to want to drink? Just as you need to do with a mapping app, you need to know your current location or the LOCALE in which you are beginning your journey.

In this case, LOCALE means **Level of Change and Life Environment.**

- How ready are you to learn how to live without alcohol?
- Where are you trying to learn how to live without it?
- What does your current living environment look like?

Levels of Change

Anyone that has been able to achieve and secure a life of sobriety had to go through levels of change that took them from not believing in the need to quit drinking to actively pursuing and achieving sustained sobriety. The exciting thing about these levels of change is they are prevalent in all forms of change.

Understanding the levels helped me first to know where I was and where I needed to go to achieve my goal of sobriety. Alcoholism researchers Carlo C. DiClemente and J.O. Prochaska, introduced a six-stage model of change to help professionals understand their clients with addiction problems and motivate them to change. The levels are:

1. Pre-Contemplation
2. Contemplation
3. Preparation/Determination
4. Action
5. Maintenance
6. Termination

Level 1: Pre-Contemplation: "My drinking is not the problem."

At the height of my 'career' as an alcoholic, and I say that purposefully, I did not believe I had a drinking problem. I enjoyed drinking and getting drunk. Everyone in my social circles drank, and we supported each other by ensuring we could access beer and liquor whenever needed. I had no intentions of changing because I did not believe (or want to believe) I had a drinking problem. Since everyone around me drank I never worried about being criticized for my drinking even if I got drunk. If a problem came up as a result of someone in the crew getting too drunk, it was quickly dismissed and laughed off over drinks the next day.

The theme for the Pre-Contemplation level is **denial**. People at this level won't proceed to the next without recognizing they have a problem and are motivated strong to make a change. A shift to the next level of change usually comes as the result of a loss so dire and painful the alcoholic recognizes a change may be the best way to avoid a genuinely unwanted outcome such as loss of freedom, physical harm to a loved one, death, etc. For me, a third DUI under the threat of jail time (among a list of other cumulative losses) caused me to finally consider a change.

Pre-Contemplation: What to consider

For someone in the Pre-Contemplation stage of change, it is vital to know a few things. Firstly, the decision to change is *yours to make*. No one else can or is responsible for ensuring you change no matter how bad they may want it or think you need it. That said, we can all benefit from exploring the possibility of knowing what we stand to gain from making changes in our lives. One can explore the possibility of change without necessarily committing to change itself. It's always good to know what you stand to gain from improving your current way of living.

How much money could sobriety pay me?

Consumption Cost Analysis

The first thing I considered was the financial implications of an alcohol-free life. I calculated how much I spent on alcohol daily. It looked like this:

On an average day, I would purchase and consume at least three tall cans of beer and a half pint of Courvoisier

Tall can price – $1.25 x3 = $3.75

½ pint of Courvoisier - $11.99

Total - $15.74 per day

$472.20 per month

$5,666.40 year

Drinking career – 1996-2011

Drinking career total = $84,996 before taxes

with 8% tax ($6,799.68) =

$91,795.68 TCC (Total Consumption Cost)

This is a *very* conservative estimate. This number does not consider increased weekend drinking at nightclub prices, birthday drinking, special occasions, all-out binges, and depressed drinking. Paying for other people's drinks is not accounted for in this example, which would quickly increase this number to over $100,000.

Calculate your current consumption cost:

Daily alcohol cost

A. $_____ per day

B. $_____ per month

C. $_____ per year

D. I have been an active drinker for _____ years

C X D = $_____ Total Consumption Cost

After looking at your calculations, consider the cost of a life of sobriety and what you can do with the money you will save in sobriety.

Level 2: Contemplation: "*I'm not saying my drinking is a serious issue but cutting down might be good for me.*"

After my first DUI, I began to quietly entertain the possibility that my drinking was getting out of hand. I had smashed up a second vehicle and started noticing an increase in losses due to my drinking. At one point, my mother and I worked at the same school; she was an on campus counselor, and I was a teacher. On Thursdays, I would go to a local club to party, socialize, and drink until 2am.

One Friday, I overslept and was late for work. I was extremely hung-over. After I looked at the clock twice and realized how late I was, I hopped out of bed and didn't even shower; I threw on clothes, washed my face briefly, and dashed out the door. I showed up to work an hour late, wreaking of alcohol so bad that my mother, who also worked at the school, caught me before anyone noticed I had entered the building. Upon smelling my breath and unwashed body said, "My God Son, you smell like a brewery! Turn around and go home now!"

I returned home and called in to say that my car had broken down and I had no way to make it to work that day. Although it would be years before I'd take my sobriety seriously, that day always stood out in my head as a day when I truly entered the next level of change: contemplation.

The Contemplation stage is where enough has happened in your life, that you consider there may be an issue with your drinking. You may not necessarily think of yourself as an alcoholic. Still, you do consider the fact that enough negative consequences have happened as a result of your drinking that you want to eliminate it from your life or at least cut it down. This is where you teeter-totter between actively addressing your addiction and letting things be.

Contemplation: What to consider

If you are in the contemplation stage, it will benefit you to think about sobriety's positive and negative aspects. After completing the Active Drinker Expense exercise, I had a clear view of how sobriety would benefit me financially. I then started thinking about the bills I could cover, the assets I could afford, and the quality of life I could attain with that money. Jay-Z once said, "Men lie, women lie, numbers don't lie." Seeing the numbers made it real for me.

What are three things you believe you could gain by living a life of sobriety?

Level 3: Preparation and Determination: I need to stop drinking, but how?

Watching my son's face as he stared at me being taken away to jail was when I knew I had to change my drinking habits. I did not want him to follow in my footsteps and become an alcoholic. The trials associated with being a Black man in America are hard enough without the added stress of dealing with the burden of alcohol addiction. That's when I chose in 2011 to stop drinking altogether. Sitting in a cell, I knew I had to fight for sobriety; I had to look at it differently than I had in the past.

At this level, you have committed to actively pursue change. This is the life-changing part of change development. This level is marked by a lot of reading on the steps one can take toward transitioning to a life of sobriety. Many people try to skip this part of the process and go straight into actively changing their behavior without a plan or knowledge of all the available resources. This can often lead to relapse. While one is passionate about making the change to addiction, it is important to get informed about resources for relapse avoidance so that they don't bounce back into old behaviors. It is crucial to consider the obstacles you will face in your fight for sobriety. World famous music producer Dr. Dre once said, "Making $1 million isn't the hard part; it's keeping $1 million that's difficult." This can also be compared to your sobriety. One may be able to attain sobriety but consistently maintaining a sober lifestyle often requires more than passion; it requires recognition of a problem and a willingness to pursue a solution in recovery.

Level 4: Action (Actively making the change)

After past attempts and a few relapses, I decided to do whatever it took to stand firm in my sobriety. I began reading literature on battling alcoholism and asking nondrinkers for advice. I thought about why I had relapsed in the past and what I could do differently to avoid repeating the same mistakes. My quest for sobriety became an addiction in itself. I started examining my spiritual beliefs, attending church regularly and connecting with my higher power. I began to focus on personal growth, feeling increasingly confident I could improve my life and never have my son know me as a drinker.

In the action stage, a person begins to feel they can change their behavior and are actively involved in taking steps to do so. This is the stage where you are most open-minded to all types of techniques and will employ them to find and define your own life of sobriety. People at this level make significant internal and external efforts to quit and change their behavior. They start developing tactics and strategies to strengthen their self-confidence. They begin creating a support system.

Your level of change speaks to your inner will and ability to pursue change. Your learning environment speaks to the outside place where this change will take place. Both must be considered and addressed for change to happen. A lemon seed must be a lemon seed to have the potential to change into a lemon tree. The ground must be fertile wet soil for that potential to manifest. Without either, the chance of transition from seed to a tree is little to none.

You will need a relapse prevention plan to move on to the next stage. Consider what you will gain and lose from a life of sobriety. I was not expecting to lose friends (aka drinking buddies) and connections to people because of sobriety, but I learned that this loss is part of the process. It is also the reason some relapse; therefore, it is vital to explore these feelings and discuss them with a trusted confidant or professional. You want to address and process these feelings to protect the life of sobriety you have worked so hard for.

Level 5: Maintenance (Actively maintaining the change)

After my first year of complete sobriety, I "came out" as a retired alcoholic. I was married to my life of sobriety, fully committed to doing everything I could never to drink again. I fought relapse with the same tenacity I used to fight to find a drink at 3 a.m. when all the bars and stores were closed. I did not want to "mess up" my sober streak and publicly let it be known that "aside from my kids, sobriety was the greatest gift God ever gave me." My sobriety was hard-earned, and I wasn't going to give it up for anything. That doesn't mean that I didn't face urges and struggles. I've suffered through the deaths of many loved ones, divorce, court, co-parenting, job losses, and financial stress, all without a drink.

In early sobriety is important to anticipate and address the things that may lead you to drink. If you relapse, you always have the opportunity to recover. You are not a failure; it is simply a speed bump on the road to change. There is only failure in giving up. You can adjust your relapse prevention plan to prepare for future obstacles.

The Wild Card: Relapse

In relapse, an individual reverts to unwanted behavior. Don't feel discouraged if you have relapsed in the past, as I did (on multiple occasions). Although 70% of people relapse within the first year of recovery, the numbers go down to less than 50%. After five years, there is only a 15% chance that you will relapse. I told myself I would consider drinking after one year without alcohol. I did this to give myself something to fight for, something to look forward to. I went from fighting for the right to have that drink in a year to fighting for my continued sobriety.

Relapse: What to consider

If you relapse it's important to remember what Winston Churchill once said, "Success is not final; failure is not fatal: it is the courage to continue that counts. You are always granted the opportunity to try again and start on day one." I did it multiple times until sobriety stuck. This is the beauty of sobriety; as long as you are blessed to remain among the living you always have the opportunity to try again with the knowledge gained from the past.

Here are a few quick assessments you can take to see if you may possibly suffer from Alcohol Dependency Syndrome according to the World Health Organization:

ICD-10 Criteria for the Alcohol Dependence Syndrome (ADS)

Three or more of the following manifestations should have occurred together for at least 1 month or, if persisting for periods of less than 1 month, should have occurred together repeatedly within a 12-month period:

- A strong desire or sense of compulsion to consume alcohol;
- Impaired capacity to control drinking in terms of its onset, termination, or levels of use, as evidenced by alcohol being often taken in larger amounts or over a longer period than intended; or by a persistent desire to or unsuccessful efforts to reduce or control alcohol use;
- A physiological withdrawal state when alcohol use is reduced or ceased, as evidenced by the characteristic withdrawal syndrome for alcohol, or by use of the same (or closely related) substance with the

intention of relieving or avoiding withdrawal symptoms;

- Evidence of tolerance to the effects of alcohol, such that there is a need for significantly increased amounts of alcohol to achieve intoxication or the desired effect, or a markedly diminished effect with continued use of the same amount of alcohol;
- Preoccupation with alcohol, as manifested by important alternative pleasures or interests being given up or reduced because of drinking; or a great deal of time being spent in activities necessary to obtain, take, or recover from the effects of alcohol;
- Persistent alcohol use despite clear evidence of harmful consequences, as evidenced by continued use when the individual is aware, or may be expected to be aware, of the nature and extent of harm. (p.57, WHO, 1993)

If that Boy Don't Swim, He's Bound to Drown!

When I was nine years old my father decided to teach me how to swim. The house I grew up in had a pool in the front yard. As a child, I would always gaze at the pool, watching my parents swim when they would have parties at the house, looking forward to the day I would learn. My father instructed me to walk down the steps at the pool's edge. Terror washed over my body as I stared into the watery abyss, feeling like I was a skydiver on the edge of a huge cliff. I paused, not knowing how the hell I was supposed to enter the pool without drowning.

My father yelled to me, "Keep going, son, get *in* the pool!" As I stood in fearful defiance, refusing to proceed, I was getting a little agitated. He told me that once I got in, he would show me all I needed to know so I could be free to swim like a fish. My attempts to whimper audibly and look as pitiful as possible to signal to my father to save me were to no avail. In a frustrated tone of finality, he said, "Son! I'm not going to say it again, Get in the pool!'"

Still refusing to enter, my father suddenly walks toward me and picks me up out of the water. Breathing a sigh of relief, I'm thinking, "Finally, my father has read me and is now going to gently…

SPLASH.

This man picked me up, held me above his head like a WWE wrestler, and threw me in the pool. (at least that's how I remember it)

I then realized that my beloved father was trying to kill me!

As an avalanche of water washed through my nostrils and mouth, I flapped my arms furiously like a newborn bird in a frantic attempt to stay afloat. My father, the navy veteran that could have easily saved me, stood at the edge of the pool, watching me fight death with a look of sadistic amusement. Trying not to laugh, he instructed me to calm my ass down and paddle. As I went to war with the water, with all the fight I could muster, I soon realized I could stand up freely in the shallow end. The water was up to my neck.

My father then entered the pool. After a short lecture on the benefits of staying calm in a crisis, my father reassured me that he wouldn't let anything happen to me. He then taught me how to float then held me up while teaching me to kick my feet. I spent the rest of the day sailing and doggy paddling; I would then join a swim team and strengthen my aquatic skills to the point where I had perfected the big four: freestyle, backstroke, breaststroke, and butterfly. Thanks to my father, I can swim like a fish to this day.

I learned something important that day about being decisive, taking initiative, and how the world works. Life has a way of putting you in a position to make decisions whether you like it or not. I could've decided to start swimming on my own terms but when the time was up my father made it clear that I no longer had any say in the matter; I was either going to start learning to swim or drown. That's it.

Once in the water, I could have started learning to swim at my own pace. Although I might have felt uncomfortable, which is natural when trying anything new, I would have been less stressed about the process because I was in full control of the situation. Although I thought my father was cruel for throwing me into the pool, I now understand why he did it and what it taught me about life.

Beginning your journey to sobriety is no different. You're not going to have all the answers when you start, but that's not what matters. What matters is making a decision and taking the first step toward sobriety.

The fact is most people don't seek sobriety until their life is facing irreparable damage. They may end up in jail where they lack access to alcohol or are threatened with termination from a job that is too valuable for them to lose. Unfortunately, many have died and are no longer among the living to drink. It is always better for you to take the initiative than to be put into a situation where quitting is your only choice. You want to walk into your sobriety with a sense of power. Making the voluntary decision to stop drinking gives you a sense of power and confidence that can be used to strengthen you on your journey.

Initiative is the necessary ingredient in every great endeavor.

The 12 Superpowers of Sobriety

When looking at the pursuit of sobriety, it is important to understand the full range of benefits that come from a life of sobriety. Alcoholics are such because they have a physical, psychological, and emotional dependence on alcohol. They feel they need it to function and deal with society and the realities of life. It has often been said that "Alcohol is a fake friend." This is true. It comes into your body using pleasure to instill a destructive dependence that can do everything from causing chemical imbalances to ending your life.

Sobriety can bring you superpowers that are not afforded to the intoxicated. As I grew in my earnest, I noticed I gained many new abilities and strengthened my traits and characteristics. Sobriety helped to supercharge personal attributes blunted by my intoxicated lifestyle. They grew to the point of being superpowers that now benefit me in all areas of my life. I believe these superpowers are afforded to all who transition from an alcoholic to an alcohol-free lifestyle. The following explains the superpowers and how they benefit you more than you'll ever know. These superpowers can affect your life and the lives of others, your loved ones, and the greater society in general.

1. The Superpower of Organic Clarity

"The eye is the lamp of the body. If your eyes are healthy, your whole body will be full of light. 23 But if your eyes are unhealthy, your whole body will be full of darkness. If then the light within you is darkness, how great is that darkness!"
-Mathew 6:22-23

According to Harold Fowler, within the context of Mathew 6:22, the eye represents an individual's guiding light, the conscience, and moral compass by which information is received, assessed, and acted upon. If the eye is sound and "clear," the information it receives is light, aka the truth, to the individual. If the eye is corrupted, dirty, or distorted (by alcohol), then what it sees will be corrupted and the acts that result from this distortion. Amid alcohol dependence our perceptions are easily distorted, and we react to these things based on the incorrect, or at best, slightly distorted vision we see. When choosing to live a life of sobriety, you are taking back the superpower of clarity that will help to inform more appropriate actions. There are many times when I reacted (or overreacted) to situations based on my skewed perception of events caused by my intoxication. The superpower of clarity will automatically strengthen your ability to make better-informed decisions.

To be completely clear, the superpower is the power of alcohol-free clarity. By this, we mean that when a former alcohol dependent becomes sober, they gain access to the power of seeing things as they are without the impediment of alcohol-infused perception. Initially, this gift can be seen as a curse, especially when forced to face past traumas or personal characteristics that may not be the most flattering. The superpower in this is that through clarity, a sober person can take life on life's terms and solve problems in a way that's rational and beneficial. Alcohol clouds judgment and makes your perception of events unclear. Alcohol is the only drug that causes an increase in aggression, which can seriously alter the perception one has of a situation. There isn't a single substance involved in more homicides than alcohol. Around 40% of convicted murderers were under the influence of alcohol when they committed their crimes. The power of clarity for someone who once never had it or lost it due to alcohol dependence is a power that is to be appreciated and respected.

2. The Superpower of Self-Reflection

Self-reflection is defined as the capacity to *exercise introspection and the willingness to learn more about one's fundamental nature and purpose.* It is usual to use the term *introspection* interchangeably with the term self-reflection because they mean more or less the same thing. Self-reflection is the opposite of external observation, which refers to the process of the individual looking outside of themselves to the physical world

The power of self-reflection can only be attained when you have a true, honest, and clear understanding of who you once were and who you want to be in the future. In an alcoholic state of mind, you have decreased control over your present and your future is questionable because you are being guided by a possession that the alcohol has over you. This is why an alcoholic's life is often chaotic and unpredictable. Once you become sober you can start to honestly reflect on your actions, true feelings, and insecurities, which may be hard but necessary for self-growth and mental health. You gain confidence and strength to move forward in all aspects of your life.

3. The Superpower of Restoration

Once alcohol-free clarity is gained the power and ability to self-reflect causes you to better appreciate the damage your past actions have caused. This is when the superpower of restoration comes into play. Step nine in the 12-step program for Alcoholics Anonymous, those working the program are advised to make direct amends for all the wrongdoings that they've committed in their addiction. This can only be done in a sober mind state. With clarity, you can objectively look at your past life and see where you have wronged others, then take the first step towards restoring relationships with others that may have otherwise been ruined.

4. The Superpower of Self-Possession

Self-possession is a vehicle of self-control. It is an ability to decide for oneself that is honest and pure of heart. Self-possession keeps you sober and what it takes to get back to that life if you relapse. This power becomes a superpower for the sober because alcohol is what you gave yourself to in the past. Alcohol is where your decisions come from, and alcohol plays a major part in the negative decisions. Once you gain the superpower of self-possession, you also begin to make choices with honest, clear intentions.

5. The Superpower of Atonement

The ability to atone for intoxicated actions of the past can only be gained through sobriety. Although you may have had drunken apologetic rants that were reflective of your true heart, the act does not reflect an intention to change. It is lip service. Thus, apologizing while drunk is not worthy of true atonement because it is not you that is apologizing with honest intention to change your behavior. You are not speaking from the heart; you are speaking from the bottle. The Superpower of atonement is that people who receive this gift are witnessing your honesty not just through words but through your behavior. Even if they don't forgive you, you can begin to heal by forgiving yourself, knowing that you did everything you could to show genuine remorse and doing what you can to change for the better to avoid repeating the same mistakes of the past.

6. The Superpower of Elimination (The Power to Go to War with Your Iniquities)

"Know thyself, and you win the battle" *Sun Tzu.*

As you gain clarity, atone for intoxicated actions of the past, and seek restoration, you will be in a stronger position to address personal flaws that come from you outside of your alcohol dependence. Maybe you're a narcissist; perhaps you are too easily angered, which can lead you to drink. Maybe you are chronically codependent on people that are part of a negative crowd or suffer from low self-esteem? Through consistent sobriety, all of these issues will reveal themselves because you are no longer using alcohol consumption to avoid them. This superpower allows you to put together an effective plan for change.

7. The Superpower of Attraction

I have never met a sober person who looked worse than they did when living as an alcoholic. Anybody who has met somebody who has gained their sobriety can attest that they physically look better. Your discipline will give you self-confidence that will radiate and be attractive to others.

Those around you that used to drink with you and secretly wish they could end their addiction to alcohol will gain strength from you. You will attract others seeking to find out how you did it. On my sober journey, I've had multiple people from my past who knew me when I drank ask me how

I did it. My real life and recovery were evidence that I must have gained something, which is why I chose to pass on what I learned and the techniques that helped me. What helped me may not be the same techniques that would help them, but the insight I offer has given them a foundation of proven strategy on which to build.

8. The Superpower of Added Value

Your presence as a sober-minded individual automatically adds value to any group to which you belong, whether it's a sports team, a team of friends going out for the night, a platoon of soldiers going to war, or business partners. You add value to every group. Alcoholics can often be a burden, depending on others to either get you home safely or keep you from fighting because you said something crazy in a drunken stupor. Your physical, mental, and social abilities add value to your group of friends, coworkers, or any team you're on. In sobriety, you can become an asset to everyone around you.

9. The Superpower of Influence

When people seek advice and guidance, the last person they want to talk to is inebriated and cannot control themselves. Your opinions within a group may matter when you've shown the strength and ability to break your dependence on the bottle. People will know you have the power of self-reflection, the power of resolution, the power to be objective, and the power to reconcile yourself, which in turn gives you the power to help others reconcile with themselves. Your input in discussions, thoughts, and opinions are focused and therefore more respected by others.

10. The Superpower of Temperance

Temperance is the ability of self-restraint. Back in the day, the anti-alcoholic movement was called the temperance movement, but in this context, the superpower of temperance is meant to mean the superpower of self-restraint and balance. The fact that you're able to remain sober means you are restrained from drinking alcohol. This temperance is a power that starts with your self-restraint from alcohol but can also lead to restraint in other areas of your life. For many of you, when you drink, you would also start smoking. For me, marijuana and liquor went together. Once I stopped drinking liquor, I noticed that my marijuana use also declined. I cannot be honest with you and say that I have completely stopped smoking marijuana, but I can say that it is not something I abuse. That Superpower is a direct result of my temperance with alcohol. As you live a consistently sober life, you will find that you'll become more mindful of what you put in your body, your emotions will be more controlled, you'll get in fewer fights, and you'll become a more positive person.

11. The Superpower of Your Position In The Universe

With sobriety comes clarity unlike no other. One of the clearest thoughts you will find as you get deeper and deeper into the beautiful life of sobriety is your defined position on this planet. Your purpose becomes clear. The reason you are here begins to formalize as a result of the clear mind and thoughtful actions you take on your road to sobriety and maintenance thereof. You will find new passions, pursue new things, and learn new things in active sobriety. I have learned that my story is what I was sent here to bring and why I wrote this book, and it is why I love doing what I'm doing. Sobriety put me in a position to help myself and others.

12. The Superpower of Redemption

Among the Superpowers of Sobriety, the strongest and most important is the one that you never lose once you start on this road to sobriety—and that is the superpower of redemption. This power is the power to bounce back from relapse. This power is available to every single person that has ever attempted sobriety, whether you are no longer sober, whether you are drunk right now; this power will remain with you until the day they die. This is the power to try sobriety again. All the other superpowers can diminish when sobriety is lost, but the power to try again never diminishes once it is established. The attempt at sobriety can only establish it but once the effort is made the power to come back is a gift that will never leave you. It is the most vital, dependable, and loyal power you'll ever possess, for it can never be taken away.

What Brings You to the Bottle?

"In large part, alcohol doesn't attract consistent attention as a killer because it's legal, easily available, and socially acceptable. In fact, it's so deeply ingrained in our culture that not drinking in some circumstances can be perceived as out of the ordinary."

-Dr. Barbara Krantz

Director of Addiction Medicine

Caron Renaissance Treatment Center in FL

I had posted a question on Facebook for friends to answer. The question was;

When did you know you had to stop drinking ?

The following is a response by Donnell Jackson:

"I knew I had to stop drinking when I tore up a Burger King and damn near went to jail!"

-Donnell Jackson

It was New Year's Eve, 1996. I was 19 years old. Bill Clinton had been reelected for a second presidential term, Pokemon, Fox News, and Dexter's Laboratory had just been introduced to the world, and we as a nation were mourning the death of West Coast Hip-Hop icon Tupac Shakur. Although I was in the mood to party my ass off as I normally did every New Year's Eve, I had the misfortune of being scheduled to work that night at Burger King.

Although I spent that night flipping burgers for drunken partygoers on their way to and back from end of the year festivities, I was also "blessed" with a manager who, by his admission, was a functional drunk as well. After closing, he allowed the staff to engage in a little celebratory drinking to bring in the New Year.

Two 40' ounces of Olde English 800 malt liquor, a shot of Bacardi 151, and a "splash" of Hennessey and Coke later, I was a whole wreck.

Things went from 0 to 100 expeditiously once I physically assaulted the manager, tore up three chairs, and damn near threw a newspaper-dispensing unit through the store window.

Police got called, and I could have easily gone to jail, but in a display of honor (or pestering guilt), the manager took the blame for it all.

Although I avoided any personal tragedy, I must send my sincerest condolences, thoughts, and prayers out to the family of the dog I hit on the way home. I haven't sipped alcohol since Jan 1, 1997.

Fishin and Sippin'

For me, I knew I had to stop drinking when my four-year-old son watched me get arrested and taken away to jail for my third DUI.

After going on a few fishing trips in 2008, a good friend of mine and I decided to create an online video series called The Funky Fishing Show. I was the producer and my fraternity brother and good friend; Anthony "Aquaman" Taylor was the host. Anthony had a nice boat and was an avid fisherman that went out often. On the show, we would go to local lakes to fish, drink and film the great times we had. We'd film funny skits, crack jokes, and inform our audience on the proper way to catch, gut, and clean fish. Back then, fishing shows were very white, very quiet, very corny, and very boring, so we figured we would create a fishing show that was Black, hip, fun, and informative. We accomplished this with Anthony's electric personality, and my hip-hop-infused editing technique. 'Fishin and sippin' is what we did whenever we went out to shoot. Coolers on the boat stay filled with beer and bottles.

One Saturday we decided to go to the lake strictly for fun. Although I normally brought the camera out and filmed content whenever we were on the water, this trip was for enjoying time with friends and family so Anthony brought his girlfriend and I brought my wife and kids. During the trip I rarely picked up the camera, occasionally taking pictures of the lake and beautiful scenery.

After a day of hanging out on the water, we headed back to the dock. When we got to the shore, Anthony asked me to get the truck and trailer so we could hook up the boat and leave the lake. I had been drinking beer with occasional shots of tequila and was drunk as hell but quickly jumped out of the boat at the shore and headed to the parking lot to get the truck and get in line to dock the boat.

While sitting in the truck waiting in the line of cars pulling their boats out of the water, I blacked. I woke up to what appeared to be a random white guy knocking on the driver's side door, asking if I was okay. As I replied, "Yes," the immediate smell of tequila must have attacked his nostrils, and he quickly flinched and blinked in disbelief. I could literally smell the Tequila seeping out of my pores. I thought he was just a concerned citizen until he asked me if I had been drinking. It was at that point that I noticed the uniform. I instinctively said, "No, well, I had a little earlier in the day, but…". By then, it was too late.

I was instructed to turn the car off and remove the keys. My wife, son, Anthony, and his girlfriend were sitting at the bottom of the dock watching the entire interaction. The officer asked for my license and proceeded back to the cruiser behind me to run my license and the car plates.

After the inevitable failure of the sobriety test to confirm the obvious, I was handcuffed and put in the back of the police cruiser to be taken to the nearest drunk tank. At the same time, Anthony, my wife, and child jumped in the truck and hooked up the boat preparing to leave. As Anthony drove by the police cruiser I was in, he stopped to let me know to call him once I got out of jail so he could come get me. My son and I locked eyes. He then turned to his mother and asked, "Mommy, why is Baba (me) in the back of that police car?" My baby boy was confused, and my wife was embarrassed. Honestly, this was one of the worst days of my life. It was also the day I decided to change my life forever. I vowed to see to it that my children would never know me as a drinker.

There are myriad reasons why we drink: to relax, escape unpleasant thoughts, numb us to our own fears, succumb to social pressure, gain a false sense of confidence, and avoid boredom or withdrawal. We are socialized to see the negative consequences of addiction. In many sobriety programs, you may be encouraged to speak at length about the things you have lost as a result of your alcoholism. This gives the alcoholic an opportunity to reflect on the negative things that have happened in their life. The hope is that they will then be motivated to sobriety by a pure drive to avoid these consequences.

Although there is certainly credence to understanding the negative consequences and real-life losses associated with alcohol addiction, there also must be an honest understanding of motivating factors that lead us to drink, especially in a world where drinking alcohol is not only legal but promoted to the masses. We must do this to put these perceived incentives in their proper perspective. The myths behind the perceived benefits must be addressed to properly understand our motivation to drink and how we can eliminate the need to drink from our lives.

Defining your "whys" for drinking

1. Physical Incentives: The feel-good elixir

It is essential to think about how alcohol makes you feel. An alcoholic is not just addicted to the liquor itself; they are also addicted to the change in state that comes with alcohol consumption. The positive benefits of being drunk need to be identified with the understanding that the same feeling can be accomplished by less dangerous means. These feelings can also be replaced by other feelings—better feelings, but you must know what you get out of it before you can seek the replacement. Does alcohol make you feel physically stronger? Relaxed? Does it help you maintain an erection? Distract you from inner pain? Be honest with yourself when assessing these benefits because many times they are what will drive you back to relapse without resolution.

2. Psychological Incentives: Liquid Courage, Confidence, Invincibility

Alcohol alters your mental state. There are psychological changes and perceptions that are attached to overdrinking. One thing alcohol gave me was a false sense of confidence. Apprehensions I might have about approaching women or dealing with interpersonal situations were all cast aside as soon as I had enough alcohol in me. In high school, before I ever drank, I was a naturally outgoing person, naturally confident, and naturally optimistic. I had no problem making friends, joking, or approaching and holding conversations with new people. As I grew up and was socialized to add alcohol to my life, I began to depend on alcohol to achieve the same social assertiveness I had as a teenager. This is a confidence that I still work to attain to this day. I always remind myself of a time before alcohol when I was just as willing to take risks without the need for alcohol.

3. Social Incentives: Alcohol as a social glue
(Jarrod Collier @strengthintime)

"I was always a cool kid growing up, but I often did outlandish things while drunk and high when amongst my friends. A friend of mine once said that while alcohol and drugs are bad for humans they often serve as a type of "social glue". Alcohol and drugs often bring groups of people together. People get together and drink or do drugs as a means to lose their inhibitions and then enjoy each other's company. This then becomes a part of the group's functional identity. It became my identity. I was the Party Guy, the guy that would set the party off while drunk or high. Unfortunately for me, the party never stopped. After high school, while my friends were preparing to go off to college, I worked for the weekend—to party and support my addiction.

At age 19, while getting drunk with friends, playing poker, and losing money, a friend dumped some cocaine on the table. That was when I became not only an alcoholic but also a drug addict. My depression grew the more I drank and used to the point where I no longer wanted to live. I was not only using but also selling drugs until I got locked up. On August 13[th,] 2013, I got as drunk as possible and started going to different bars to say goodbye to my friends, as I had planned on killing myself that evening.

After a day of visits, I got home, dumped a mass of pills in my hand, and took them intending never to wake up again. Fortunately, I passed out before taking a fatal dose. I woke up in a hospital. When I woke up, I was surprisingly relieved to be alive. I heard a voice speak to me and tell me that I had been granted a second chance at life. At that moment, I decided to be done with drugs and alcohol.

Unlike hard drugs, alcohol is woven within the fabric of world culture. In America, there isn't a sport show, music program, or pop culture event that is void of some type of liquor promotion. You can name plenty movies where a character died from a drug overdose but would be hard pressed to find one where a main character died because of drunk driving or alcohol poisoning.

Everyone has a desire to be liked, loved, and favored. No one really cares to be seen as socially awkward or a social burden to the group. Liquor can erode inhibitions that cause us to focus on these things. This byproduct of "confidence" in doing what everyone else is doing feels good. When drinking with others, buying drinks for other people, and becoming drunk with others builds a comradery that one can begin to depend on, and feel is impossible to reach without alcohol.

As Robert Schuller suggests, "Success is never ending, failure is never final." Celebrate the fact that unlike many others, you have now taken the first step on the path to sobriety, you have begun by making a choice to pursue it.

Step 2: LEARN

"Education becomes more relevant once you know what you want to do with it."
-Vusi Thembeckwayo

The Addiction:

"Proper perspective precedes powerful planning." – Hanief Saterfield

An alcoholic is an addict because they do not know how to avoid overdrinking. They don't know how to live without alcohol. They don't know how to see themselves as a non-drinker. Many alcoholics also don't know why they need to stop drinking when it seems like others can "handle their liquor" just fine, so why can't they? Without addressing these reasons, it will be very difficult to live a sober life.

Medical News Today defines the word 'addiction' as: "A psychological and physical inability to stop consuming a chemical, drug, activity, or substance, even though it is causing psychological and physical harm."

Although this may be the given definition, I believe words have a power that cannot be underestimated. I also believe that words establish perspective. To beat alcoholism, I had to first admit I had a problem but also know that I had the power to solve it. This required gaining an empowered perspective on my situation. Considering my alcoholism to be an inability to stop drinking means that I do not have the power to stop. I needed to believe that I had the ability to do so to live a sober life. It is for this reason that I work from the following definition of addiction:

"An addiction is a habit you are actively committed to regardless of effect or outcome."

You'll notice I have replaced the word "inability" with the word "commitment" because a commitment can be ended and is not permanent. It also reflects the fact that active addiction is a choice, not some uncontrollable part of my character that is impossible to change or conquer. For instance, you may depend on a job you hate for your food, shelter, and lifestyle. Without the job, you may suffer, yet you still have a choice to leave it. You could quit or retire from that job but you choose to stay even though it may have a negative effect on your physical or mental well-being. As such, you also have the choice to retire from a life of active alcoholism.

Retirement from alcohol abuse, just like a job, is a choice one must make for themselves. Although you may retire from a specific profession or position, you can always decide to "go back to work". As such, you can choose to 'retire' from drinking but are always able to 'come out of retirement' and go back to drinking. What helps you stay away from these past 'occupations' depends on you and the life you create for yourself upon 'retirement' in recovery.

Gaining a proper perspective of my alcohol addiction was the first thing I had to understand to arm myself with the strength to work toward sobriety. I was addicted to the habit of drinking. I was dedicated to the "job" of being drunk. Once I made the choice to retire for good I began to take up new occupations including; Health nut, gym rat, recovery coach and author. I have my sobriety to owe for all of these new, much more honorable titles and occupations. Just like being addicted to a substance or action, you can become addicted to the practice of sobriety by retiring from active alcoholism for good, building, and enjoying the new life you create for yourself.

Chart your addiction to track your recovery

Elvin Morton Jellinek (1890–1963), one of the most influential personalities in the field of alcohol studies, came up with the basis for what would soon be called the Jellinek Curve. It is an illustration that shows the phases of alcohol addiction and recovery. It lays out physical and mental characteristics familiar to anyone who has dealt with alcoholism. Take a look at the chart and try to identify where you think you are. The loop at the bottom of the chart, *The Drinker's Loop,* is the "bottom" stage where most of your career as an alcoholic dwells, before deciding to pursue sobriety. If you are there, it is imperative that you end this cycle, as this is where most either escape or stay until they die.

Below is a chart that maps a common progression for someone that falls into the trap of alcoholism. It is informed by the Jellinek Curve. As you read the list, note the steps that pertain to your experience and note your current situation based on your place on the chart.

o Started as an occasional drinker, drinking for fun, relaxation or an escape
o Relief drinking increases and dependency grows
o Alcohol tolerance increases. You need more alcohol to get the same high
o Increase in "drunk days" You start losing track of time while drinking
o Family or friends express concern
o Work and money effected by drinking

- You feel like you're the only one with this problem and don't discuss it with anyone.
- You start having blackouts
- Try to quit but fail
- Start avoiding family members and friends
- Increased drinking with other chronic drinkers
- Binging occurs
- Obsessive drinking
- Feeling guilt for use
- Thinking becomes impaired
- You know you drink too much but can't seem to stop
- Feelings of complete defeat

The Drinker's Loop

Trigger Habit Result

Addictions are based on habits. To eliminate the habit of drinking, the it must first be examined and understood. In his book *The Power of Habit,* Charles Duhigg describes the four steps of habit formation: **cue, craving, response, and reward**. All four steps are part of the drinking habit all alcoholics succumb to.

Duhigg notes that within the four-part process, only one step needs to be changed: the response. There will always be cues and a craving to achieve a change in state, but different responses can lead to the desired state. As a teacher, my drinking habit went like this: I went to work, came home felt the need to relax (cue), started longing for a drink (craving), would fix myself a glass or buy a beer on the way home (response), then feel at ease as I started on my path toward drunkenness (reward). The cue triggers the craving to drink, which is then addressed and satisfied through drinking. This habit loop occurred every day after work regardless of my mood because the routine was a self-perpetuating cycle. It became as unconscious as going to the bathroom when I had a full bladder.

According to James Clear in his book, *Atomic Habits*, what we crave is not the alcohol, but the change in the mental state the alcohol delivers to us, a physical and mental divergence from our current reality. We crave the feeling the alcohol provides us. Think about the steps that lead you to drink, and you will find that there is always a cue that leads to the craving and a state change you are working to achieve through drinking. Defining your drinking habit loop will help you uncover a process for change.

When I chose sobriety, I replaced the drinks I used to have after work with a light snack, a walk around the block, or a good workout. This made me feel better and gave me the same similar type of 'high' I used to get from alcohol. My fitness began to affect my confidence. It changed how I saw others and how I saw myself. Also, exercise releases dopamine, the "pleasure chemical" released when you take drugs or drink. I realized that after working out for a couple months, my sobriety started to show in my skin and physique. My skin was clearing up and new muscle started replacing fat deposits left by years of drinking. This motivated me to replace my drinking with working out consistently. My new response gave me something that alcohol couldn't, better physical health.

The Drinker's Jacket: Changing your Social Identity

"The lens through which others see you that becomes how you see yourself..."

As we descend into alcoholism, we develop an identity that permeates our lives in addiction.

Parts of your individual identity that are affected by sobriety

- Physical identity - How we look
- Behavioral identity - How we act
- Social identity - How we interact with others

The transition to sobriety will include changes in all areas of your identity: your physical, behavioral, and social identity. Once you stop drinking, your body begins healing itself because it doesn't have to expend the energy required to process heavy amounts of alcohol. You will be sober-minded, making you sharper and more in control of your behavior. You will begin to act in a manner that is truer to yourself. You will also be able to start working on the issues that led you to drink.

Most people applaud the physical and behavioral changes that come with sobriety but can be resistant to a change in your social identity. I had a challenging time dealing with social identity in sobriety. This is because your social identity is who you are to yourself and others. It is your "jacket." When your social identity is alcohol-centered it becomes what I call your "Drunk Jacket."

A 'jacket" refers to a prisoner's file which contains all information on a prisoner. This file is used to establish the reputation by which other inmates judge an inmate. An inmate with a 'snitch jacket' has evidence in his paperwork that he has testified against a codefendant or another criminal in return for reduced time or some other personal benefit. Once an inmate is seen as having a snitch jacket he is forever judged by and treated as a snitch regardless of how he conducts himself in the future. It is a label that sticks eternally. Your jacket is the lens through which others see you.

The 'Drunk Jacket': How your alcoholism becomes your identity

The 'drunk jacket' is the term I use to describe alcohol-centered social identity. It is a jacket that is not only earned by an alcoholic's excessive drinking but also by actions associated with their excessive drinking.

Although no one cares to be considered an alcoholic and wear a drunk jacket there is a process we go through which takes an alcoholic from being resistant to the label to becoming comfortable with the label to the point of actively promoting the alcoholic lifestyle to others. As an alcoholic, it is the process by which your addiction becomes your identity.

Denial	You reject the drunk jacket
Acceptance	You accept your drunk jacket
Promote	You promote your drunk jacket
Protection	You protect your drunk jacket

First, you deny this social identity. You may say things like "I may drink a lot but I'm not an alcoholic!" With time and experience, you soon begin to accept the jacket because you hang around others with the same jacket who are often unapologetic about their addictive tendencies. Next, you protect your social identity by making sure you have access to alcohol wherever you are. Lastly, you get to the point where you promote your jacket in thought, speech, and action.

When I was first accused of being an alcoholic, I rejected it because I felt I was in control of my drinking and didn't like the stigma of powerlessness that came with being called an alcoholic. In other words, I was lying to myself. At that time, I considered myself a heavy drinker because it was a more acceptable title. After a while, I no longer resisted the alcoholic reputation. I started gravitating toward other alcoholics; just about everyone in my circle was either an alcoholic or a daily drinker. Whenever we got together, the first thing we did was get drunk. It was the tie that bound us together. If we were without alcohol for too long, we would come together to work on getting more. Our relationships were dependent and predicated on the presence and consumption of alcohol. This part of addiction must be addressed and planned for if you want any *real* hope of staying sober.

It has been said that social group memberships inform our self-concept. In a sense, "who I am" is partially determined by "who we are." Other alcoholics in our social group often influence our perception of our lives of addiction. We initially resist the identity, only to self-identify as a drinker, stoner, or junkie without shame. This is what makes the Drinker's Jacket so dangerous. For many socially isolated people, their connection and dependence on their addict group is even stronger.

Here are a few reasons why it is often hard to change your social identity:

1. Your alcoholic social ID is comfortable (It is what you know and what you're used to)
2. Everyone knows you this way. (Your friends and family are used to this version of you no matter how much they do or don't like it.)
3. This identity holds many memories, both positive and negative.

4. Often, many people around you share the same addiction or social identity

An inability to deal with social identity change is a common reason for many who relapse. Humans often return to the role they are most comfortable with—especially when facing adversity. Knowing this, it is crucial to take steps to establish a social identity that is not attached to your addiction. You must take off the Drinker's Jacket. There are a few things you can do to start working on upgrading your social identity as you move into recovery.

How to upgrade your social identity:

1. **Define** your ideal self: "Who are you growing to become?"
2. **Understand** the connection between your sobriety and your personal growth. How will sobriety help you become a better version of yourself?
3. **Analyze** the social challenges you face against your old identity. Who and what are the people and things that challenge your sobriety the strongest? How can you address these challenges?

4. **Control** your conversations to focus on wins and solutions (Don't "wallow in the mire")

The goal of the above exercise is to help *empower your view of yourself* in sobriety.

Sobriety Reaction Types

People will react to your newfound sobriety in different ways. Many people who first start on their journey to lifelong sobriety are surprised to find that many of the reactions to their sobriety aren't as positive as they had expected. Surely those who know and love you, your friends and family, would be ecstatic at the news of your newfound sobriety. Right?

While discussing this with Kela, a college friend, she talked about how surprised she was surprised at some of the reactions she got from her own family when she told them about her pursuit of sobriety. Some of her cousins stopped talking to her altogether. They told her she was bound to relapse and asked her why she would stop drinking completely when she could just moderate. Your friends and family are all used to and comfortable with you being the alcoholic they have grown to know and expect regardless of the negative consequences that drinking had in your life. The clarity she gained from this experience showed she had many friends and relatives who loved her as long as she was a drunk mess but saw her as a threat to their insecurities on her road to sobriety.

Some of your old drinking partners may inadvertently or purposefully try to get you to relapse so you can re-join the social group. Some may see your attempt at sobriety as an affront to their drinking lifestyle. Your choice to remain sober may trigger various reactions from friends and family. So, how do you respond in a way that protects your sobriety?

Resentment – According to Chapter Five of the *Big Book of Alcoholics Anonymous*, Resentment is the "number one" offender, referring to resolving the resentment you may have for others while recovering. However, I am referring to the resentment you will face from old drinking buddies and people closest to you that are resistant to your sobriety.

Those that resent your sobriety are usually engaged in the same addiction you are attempting to overcome and see your attempt at sobriety as an affront to their character. They will ask you why you are choosing to quit, not to gain understanding but to offer counterpoints to your reasoning.

These types are enemies to your sobriety and should be avoided if possible. If this is not possible, it will be important to prepare for their efforts to break your sobriety.

Ideal response: Let them know you are doing it for yourself and that they are free to do what they want with their own lives. No further explanation is needed because they won't be accepted anyway.

You must not seek validation from others, as that is a form of codependency. Therefore, sobriety must be 100% *your choice*. This resentfulness can manifest differently, but the goal is to convince you to relapse.

Pity – You will come across people with good intentions who treat you like a wounded lamb. They might go out of their way to hide their drinks when you come around or constantly ask you if you are okay around them while they drink. Others may be your former drinking partners, making you feel guilty about burdening them with your sober presence. They may send hints that you're killing the vibe. This form of peer pressure says more about them than you. Reverse psychology reflects their feelings of inadequacy because although they know they too should show more self-restraint (because usually, they are alcoholics), they don't have the strength to pursue sobriety. This can be difficult initially, but just like being teased, the attempts will stop if you don't respond to it.

Shame – "Don't be a bitch! You're grown, just moderate!" - These people want to make you feel weak for admitting that you have a problem with alcohol, as they usually share the same weakness. To other alcoholics, you are a mirror that many cannot face.

Although ending a life of gang banging is positive because it's safer for yourself and the community, the people in your gang will resist the idea of you no longer engaging in the illegal activity associated with gang banging. It is the same way with your drinking buddies. Often, an alcoholic's peer group will be filled with other alcoholics and or other heavy alcohol drinkers. Once the tie of alcohol consumption is removed from the relationship, the relationship loses value in the eyes of alcoholics. This is why reactions to this change in your life can often be more negative than positive. To combat this pressure and shame, you must build a community of support, a network of people conducive to your new life of sobriety.

Helping your friends adjust to your sobriety

Changing your jacket means changing how you view yourself and resisting the temptation to return to your old ways. Countless people in the Black community get a nickname attached to them that they don't like which becomes accepted by the receiver over time. The drunk jacket can be the same without resistance. Changing this jacket requires the strength to be consistent in knowing who you are or wish to be, which is a non-drinker.

People get comfortable seeing you in a particular light, whether positive or negative. Most won't admit it, but a significant change for the better is equally as uncomfortable for your peers as a negative change because it means they will have to change how they interact with you. This is a rarely discussed but major part of the reason why people relapse. Your "jacket," whether good or bad, is familiar to your peers, who have come up with ways to interact with you that they are now comfortable with. When you change, there is not only a sense of disbelief but also discomfort that your friends will have to deal with as they adjust to the new, sober you. Most of the time, your peer group shares your addiction, so your change may be taken as a negative reflection on them. Imagine a hardened criminal that goes to jail finds the Lord, no longer engaging in crime but is released to a peer group of criminals. They may have difficulty adjusting to this person who is no longer linked to them through crime.

The Fitness Analogy: A Tool for framing perspective

Even after I gained the strength and discipline to be around my drinking friends without succumbing to the urge to drink, I noticed many were still apprehensive about drinking around me. I could tell they were holding back from enjoying drinks and could not have fun around me. Honestly, I can't blame them. Although I appreciated that their choices were well intentioned and done out of care for me, I didn't want to suffer the burden of feeling like my presence was hindering others. Many don't understand how that guilt can lead some back to the bottle. To feel comfortable in my sobriety, I knew I had to be able to function among those who drink. Although I am always available to help anyone interested in living alcohol-free, I am in no way trying to preach the gospel of sobriety or force others to come with me. To protect my sobriety, I wanted to find a way to make others comfortable with it, regardless of whether or not they chose to drink around me. I developed a way to help them understand my perspective on drinking in a way that made them feel comfortable living as they pleased. I call it the *Fitness Analogy.*

Imagine a gym room full of people of different ages and sizes all there to get healthy, more substantial, etc. You've got short people, tall people, men, women, professional bodybuilders, and soccer moms who want to shed a few pounds as part of their New Year's resolution. In this gym, you have many different people with differing levels of strength: some can bench 40 lbs., 100 lbs., some 400 lbs. Some never touch a weight but choose to do cardio on the elliptical or swim in the pool because they may have bad joints, an injury, or a debilitating condition. Now think of the weights as different types of alcohol. Just because I can't lift 400lbs doesn't necessarily mean that the 400-pound weights should be removed from the building. In this analogy, I am the guy with lousy wrist joints that must find another way to strengthen myself. In a club, I would not drink to have fun, but that doesn't mean there aren't other things I can do to enjoy myself. I can dance, laugh at those that choose to get drunk, socialize with the ladies, or just chill and observe the scenery. I do not need to stop others from doing their "work out" their way. There's no shame in being at the 100lb bench or only doing cardio because you have bad joints. Everyone is different, and that's okay.

Discovering your "Why?"

The following are two stories from friends who discovered their why and decided to stop drinking.

The Crutch and the Cheerleader

(CA Henderson, MA. Ed; Author of *The Life, Victor Valley to West Point, and The 100-Day Journal Challenge*)

I knew I had to stop drinking when I had a subconscious need, want, and desire to be drunk all the time, supported by the crutch and the cheerleader. In reflection, as a person that has accepted alcoholism and the effects of alcoholism, the subconscious dependence on alcohol is the worst part of all. In explaining this, let me introduce the crutch and the cheerleader. Alcohol, and its importance in your life as a coping mechanism, is represented by the crutch who's always there to lean on and the cheerleader who is always there to cheer you on!

The ever-so-supportive crutch, always there to lean on, will never fail you. The crutch will always come through to show you support through death, difficulty, and delay. And in doing this, you remain numb, in denial, and far from present in most situations in life. I realized this critical point when a therapist suggested that I put the bottle down as I went through the grieving process of my dad's death. She wanted to ensure that I took on this difficult task with a clear mind and without the help of alcohol. In alcoholism, you always rely on the enemy for support.

The ever-so-congratulatory cheerleader is always there to cheer you on in times of happiness and joy. Winning the big game, landing the dream job, and life's most precious moments are always welcomed by the cheerleader who helps you celebrate the good times when days are good. If it's a celebration, the cheerleader is your favorite person to have with you to encourage and keep you celebrating at a high level. In alcoholism, you always rely on the enemy to cheer you on.

Alcoholics use alcohol every day. If you're not using alcohol as a crutch during the hard times, you're using alcohol as a cheerleader and then during the good times. And all the while, the enemy is consistently in your day-to-day undertakings.

Convertible Crush: Kela's Story

Kela Williams-Collins – Social Worker

"I knew I had to stop drinking after two DUIs, some jail time, and almost losing my life after flipping my convertible and landing upside down in a ravine."

In March of 2006, I was arrested for my first DUI. Exactly one year later, in March of 2007, I was arrested again for DUI and placed on 18 months probation. During my tenure as an alcoholic, it seemed that I was going for employee of the decade for the 2000s. After the traumatizing inconvenience of dealing with the courts during my first DUI, I made the drunken decision to act like the second one didn't happen and failed to appear in front of the judge. (I know, genius, right?)

About six months later, while attending my son's football game, my car was towed for parking in a handicapped spot without a sticker. Was I handicapped? No, although mentally, I could have easily argued that I had somehow forfeited the common sense offered to all of God's people.

When I went to the tow yard to pick up my car, the police didn't meet me there, they beat me there. They greeted me with a warrant and handcuffs.

This led to a two-week stay in an Orange County jail for the latest DUI before being extradited to Los Angeles' most infamous Twin Towers for a two-week stay for a violation of probation on the first DUI. Did I stop drinking? I wish I could say yes, but I'd be lying. It would take a little more than some jail time to set me on the right track.

In 2013, I moved to Texas. As an LA girl, I missed the action and California sunshine but needed to move closer to my mother as she was getting older. She lived in Greenville, which was too rural for me plus, Greenville is a semi-dry town, so moving there wasn't even an option in my mind. The closest liquor store was 20 minutes away in the college town of Commerce, and there were no jobs in my field, so I worked and lived in Desoto, where I could drink at will and still make the trip to see my mother.

While visiting my mother's house, I finished off the stash of liquor I'd typically take with me. In Greenville, they only sell beer and wine, so I had to go to the next city over to get liquor. In a drunken stupor, I took that late-night drive into the rural abyss searching for liquor in Commerce. I took my chances, traveling down a dimly lit two-lane road late at night in search of my fix. Beer and wine weren't going to work for me. I needed something with a lot more "octane" than 5% alcohol.

All seemed well on my trip until I blacked out, and the next thing I knew was upside down in a creek with my convertible crushed and half of my body hanging outside the busted car window. I had a terrible headache and had landed in brush from the dry creek bed. After being removed from the car by the paramedics, a half hour later, my mom arrived to see her daughter, shaken but alive. My car was crushed like a beer can, with the only opening on the driver's side, where I was found semi-coherent. When my mother saw the damage, she broke down and cried, thinking about how close she came to losing her only daughter.

It was at that moment that I knew something *had* to change.

Admittedly, I have relapsed a few times since then but continue to fight the good fight for my sobriety. I want to give a special shout-out to the paramedics that saved me, my therapist, my AA family, and the few genuine friends and family members that love and support me through it all."

Why do you want to stop drinking?

You were not born an alcoholic; you became one. This means that there was a time in your life when you lived without ever consuming alcohol. You had fun, met new people, and developed meaningful relationships with others without the help of alcohol. Although you may have been very young at the time, the fact remains, you lived without alcohol and, therefore, can get back to doing it again.

One way to think about your why is by conducting a cost-benefit analysis. What do you lose in your current alcoholic state versus if you were sober? List these losses and establish a two-sentence response that answers the question, "Why do you want to stop drinking." It may be for health reasons, psychological, physical, mental, or emotional reasons, or it may be for legal reasons (one more DUI meant jail time for me).

If you are having trouble articulating your "why," here are two things to think about:

1. Are you dependent?

It's not just about alcohol use. The question is, are you alcohol dependent? If you ever succumb to the *need* to have a drink, then you are, to some degree, alcohol dependent. There is nothing that alcohol gives you that you cannot get without it. It only takes away by establishing a craving, which turns into dependence. Check out the Chemical Dependency checklist below SOURCE

Chemical Dependency Checklist

C	Do you ever attempt to *conceal* your habit from others
H	Do you ever think about getting *help* for your habit
E	Do you have problems at your place of *employment* because of your habit
M	Do you ever experience a loss of *memory* as a result of your habit
I	Do you ever become severely *intoxicated*
C	Do you ever fear unfairly *criticized* because of your habit
A	Do you ever feel your habit is *abnormal*
L	Do you ever *lose* friendships or leave relationships as a result of your habit
L	Do you ever *lower* your intake you end up returning to your previous level
Y	Do you ever neglect your *young* children or other loved ones because of your habit

D   Do you become *defensive* or argumentative about your usage

E   Do you fail to get in touch with your *emotions* because of your usage

P   Is your *physical* health affected by your usage

E   Do you *enjoy* only functions were alcohol or other drugs are available

N   Is your *need* for the substance affecting your finances

D   Do you *deny* that you experience any consequences from your habit

E   Do you *evade* difficult situations by indulging in your habit

N   Is your *need* to feed your habit affecting your relationships

T   Is your *tolerance* level for the substance getting higher

If you answer **yes** to *__five or more__* of the above questions you may have a serious dependency

2. Do You Have Presence of Mind

When you lose your presence of mind it is hard to understand the concept of time and place. This is why many people get drunk and do things that are inappropriate at a given moment. They may cuss in a church or yell in a library or throw up on a nightclub dance floor and not understand the implications of their actions. If you have a drinking problem these lapses are some of the clearest red flags that have let you know that you have a problem. Crashing your car, passing out while driving, fighting for no legitimate reason, and arguing with a loved one are all lapses of the presence of mind.

The desire for social acceptance can cause us to do things we would not normally do just to fit in. No one wants to be the "odd man out" and although our likelihood of succumbing to peer pressure decreases as we get older, we can still become victims of social conditioning. Many people are encouraged by their own family to have their first drink on their 21st birthday as a "rite of passage". This sends a negative message to children by indirectly telling them that drinking is the 'grown up' thing to do as opposed to calling it what it really is, another poison that is simply acceptable to do and marketed to those 21 and older to make others rich.

There was a time when you did not need alcohol to attain these things. Alcohol itself made you a dependent. You have been dependent for so long that you see no other way to acquire these things without it. The confidence given to you by alcohol is temporary and fake. Alcohol takes away your inhibitions, which you think translates into courage. It really is just carelessness. Alcohol causes you to care less about the consequences of your actions. While carelessness and audacity can benefit you in some respects, they can also lead to detrimental outcomes in many situations, especially when mixed with another thing you lose with alcohol use, your presence of mind.

Alcohol Ugly: The symptoms

The physical effects of alcoholism often go unnoticed to the alcoholic. Over time, there are common physical maladies that occur with excessive alcohol use. I call it, becoming "Alcohol Ugly"; symptoms include:

- Dry skin – Alcohol dehydrates skin. Alcoholics RARELY drink water, which compounds the dehydration. It is one of the giveaways that someone has relapsed that you can see but might not be able to describe.
- Weight gain – It is a well-known fact that alcohol is full of "empty calories" meaning they have no nutritional value. Alcohol also causes weight gain because it reduces the amount of fat your body burns for energy. This weight usually settles in the most unwanted places on your body: your face, stomach, and sides (love handles). This is what the term "beer belly" alludes to. For my skinny ladies trying to put on some "good" weight, drinking in attempts to get "thick" will not work out the way you might hope.
- Drinking alcohol reduces the amount of fat our bodies burns for energy. While we can store nutrients, protein, carbohydrates, and fat in our bodies, we can't store alcohol, so our systems want to get rid of it, and this takes priority. All other processes that should be taking place (including absorbing nutrients and burning fat) are interrupted.

- Red eyes - Alcohol causes the tiny blood vessels in our eyes to expand, which pushes more blood to flow through them, leaving them looking bloodshot. Alcoholism take the 'bright' out of your eyes.
- Aged eyes - Arcus senilis is a gray or white arc visible above and below the outer part of the cornea — the clear, domelike covering over the front of the eye. Eventually, the arc may become a complete ring around the colored portion (iris) of your eye. Arcus senilis is a visible sign of aging and Research has shown that people who drink heavily have a 33% greater chance of getting arcus senilis, a telltale gray ring around their corneas before they turn 60. Irreversible
- Red face - heavy drinking can cause permanent facial redness. Yes, even in Black folks.
- Body Odor - Although the liver processes most of the alcohol you consume, a portion of it leaves the body directly through your breath, sweat and urine, all of which can result in an unpleasant odor.

Step 3: ACT

"I prayed for freedom for twenty years, but received no answer until I prayed with my legs."
— *Frederick Douglass*

Once you have learned about alcoholism and have determine that you wish to live a life of sobriety it is time to act. You, and only you, can make the choice to bless yourself with a life upgrade of this magnitude. Actor Rob Lowe once said, "A person cannot become sober for their wife, kids, family, or anyone else, they can only become sober once they have had enough." You have to no longer be willing to tolerate the consequences that come with an alcoholic lifestyle. You must be fed up and ready to live the life you deserve. I hit rock bottom when my son had to watch me get carted away to jail in the back of a police car. To be handcuffed and caged in the back of the police car while in front of my son was the epitome of shame for me. I never again wanted to let alcohol put me in such a position in my life.

July 24th 2011 was my first day without a drink and I have not drank since. This day is what I consider the birthday of my sobriety. Whatever day you choose to stop drinking will be your date. There are a couple things that make this day very beautiful; Firstly, it is the first day of sober life and secondly, it is the day you earn a lifelong gift, the most important of the 12 Superpowers of Sobriety, the one that can never be taken away even in relapse, **The Superpower of Redemption**.

You may be saying to yourself, "Haven't I already started taking action just by reading this book and learning about my loop and addiction patterns." Technically, yes but there are two things to consider; Firstly, you could have still been drinking during the first two steps, as you needed to assess whether pursuing sobriety was needed and if you were ready to make a conscious effort toward a life of sobriety. There is a very specific act I am referring to, an act that makes everything including your decision to live a sober life official and that act is stopping!

This is where you seal your commitment to sobriety by consciously and deliberately not drinking. Officially, you are not choosing paralysis by analysis; trying to figure out how you're going to guarantee that you will never drink again because guarantees are impossible. You are about to free yourself from the fear of failure that may have stopped you from beginning earlier. You have learned enough to make the decision to stop and therefore do it. You can use the rest of this book to help you figure out how to prepare for future social events and reactions from those your either like or love that will need to adapt to the improved, sober you.

Handling H.A.T.E.

(High Addiction Triggering Elements)

One thing we must all deal with is what I call HATE. In the realm of sobriety, I am speaking of High Addiction Triggering Elements. These are the emotional, environmental, and situational factors that push you toward your addiction. Whether it be a stressful day that causes you to want to "unwind" with a drink (that usually turns into a binge), or a night out with friends that turns into a night of bad decisions and a morning hangover, these high addiction elements can be roadblocks and challenges to your sobriety that must be analyzed and addressed in order for you to live alcohol free while being able to function in everyday society. A fight for a life of sobriety without a clear understanding of High Addiction Triggering Elements that challenge your progress is highly likely to be short-lived. The following chapter will discuss addiction triggers and how you can address them.

Addiction Triggers

An addiction trigger is something that triggers you to want to run to your addiction. Whether it is alcohol, drugs, or overeating, it is a situation or emotional state that will cause you to want to engage in your addiction. It is essential to understand and know your triggers so that you can put together a plan to counter your propensity to run to your addiction. There are three types of triggers that you must take into consideration on your road to sobriety. These are emotional triggers, environmental triggers, and situational triggers.

Emotional Triggers

- Happiness
- Sadness
- Grief
- Stress
- Boredom

Emotional triggers are states of mind that lead you toward your addiction. Although just about any emotion will do, extreme feelings of these emotions have the strongest pull towards an addiction. These emotions include extreme happiness and celebration, sadness or grief, stress, anxiety, and boredom. Everyone differs, so you need to consider which emotional triggers make you more susceptible to drinking.

1. Happiness

For the alcoholic, alcohol is a necessary part of all celebratory events and thereby attached to extreme happiness. It is for this reason that pleasure becomes an emotional trigger for drinking. On a birthday or if you win the lottery or find some form of luck, the amount of dopamine rush attached to happiness can cause you to feel carefree. You begin to feel a lack of inhibition and celebratory feelings, which are permanently attached to the consumption of alcohol.

I remember once, after work, I was happy, so I started drinking as soon as work finished. I went out that night and ended up getting a DUI and being sent to jail.

It is important to recognize when you get these feelings of elation or happiness that may trigger liquor use. You must instead put yourself in celebratory systems that are void of alcohol. You also want to be around people who are less likely to drink. You may also look for other outlets for joy that can substitute for the consumption of alcohol.

2. *Sadness (grief*

Sadness is an emotion we all look to avoid. Alcohol provides an outlet for you to forget your present state of mind usually. For this reason, an alcoholic will run to alcohol when faced with extreme sadness. This, of course, can often end up in a cycle where drinking leads to even more negative outcomes that cause you to feel more pain which can lead you to the bottle, in a recurring cycle of dysfunction. Once again, it is important to reach out to people who can help you deal with the root causes of your sadness or anger. At some point, you want to be able to address these negative feelings without the use of alcohol.

3. *Stress and Anxiety*

Like sadness, stress and anger are feelings alcoholics often look to avoid through drinking. Alcohol causes us to forget our feelings and have a momentary vacation from the situations that may cause anxiety in our lives.

Working out, jogging, and focusing on some form of self-improvement are ways I deal with stress. Using your energy to focus on a solution is the quickest way to eliminate stress.

4. Boredom

Unlike the previous emotions: happiness, stress, and anger, boredom can often be the worst and most pervasive call for drinking binges. I used to have a saying when teaching that I would rather deal with a group of angry students than bored students, and that is true to this day. The main reason I prefer an angry, upset, or stressed student over a bored student is that the former has focus. A bored child has no focus; therefore, you must try and figure out how to best divert them away from counterproductive behavior with no point of reference. This can be difficult because people respond to stimuli differently.

Situational Triggers

- Holidays and Celebrations
- Weddings
- Situations of Isolation (Trips to the Laundromat)
- Funerals

Situational triggers are situations that lend themselves to your addiction. For instance, birthday parties, celebrations of any sort, weddings, and funerals are all situations that usually will trigger an addiction. For most alcoholics, all of these situations were excuses to drink.

My first relapse was on New Year's Eve, 2010, three months after I had first attempted to stop drinking. One of my friends got out of the car with a one-gallon jug full of orange juice and vodka and handed it straight to me. He was already drunk and rather forceful in his insistence that I take a swig. Although I was able to go through Thanksgiving and Christmas without a drop, I allowed myself to fall victim to my addiction. It is important to know who in your life wants you to win or lose. Be honest with yourself about these truths. You must remember that your sobriety will be offensive to people close to you, especially if they're used to engaging in the same addicting behaviors alongside you.

- **Holiday Celebrations**

Holiday celebrations can be especially difficult for a recovering alcoholic since alcohol is almost always a part of the celebration. One thing that has worked for me is always ensuring I have some form of non-alcoholic drink in my hand. At holiday celebrations and nightclubs, I always get my nonalcoholic drinks poured in a glass usually reserved for alcoholic beverages. People will subconsciously assume that you are drinking and are less likely to hand you drinks in their attempt to help you "join the festivities." In the case of practicing sobriety around drinkers, looking the part without playing the part is a tactic that has helped me stay sober and help those around me that were used to seeing me drink be at ease.

- **Weddings**

Weddings provide the perfect excuse to get drunk. It's a celebratory occasion, just about everyone's drinking (before, during, and after the wedding) and there's usually an open bar or available drink via bottles and flasks smuggled in by attendees and groomsmen.

If your friends are like mine, everyone in the wedding party is drinking and even the groom may take a sip or two to take the nervous edge off (although they may not admit it). At my own wedding, I was drinking. Although I could avoid getting completely drunk until after the ceremony, I maintained a buzz throughout the day.

- **Isolation**

I remember when I was 22 and still living with my mother. The washing machine at our house had broken. I was an active alcoholic but wasn't comfortable drinking around my mother, so I began to look forward to taking my clothes to the Laundromat. Although many would see this as a tedious chore, I loved it because it gave me an excuse to grab a drink and sip alone while waiting on my clothes to wash and dry. The liquor store was conveniently located next door to the Laundromat so getting drunk during the spin cycle was extremely easy. I would sit in my car and drink while listening to the radio. Once, I drank so much that I passed out and woke up hours later with a washer full of damp clothes. The more I descended into my alcoholism, the more I sought situations of isolation. I believe there was a shame I felt about getting drunk in front of others that made me schedule times where I could drink alone without being judged.

- **Funerals**

Funerals can be especially difficult due to the somber nature of the event. Usually, a funeral involves someone you love and were close to. This lends itself to drinking to numb the pain of loss. You must find the strength to resist relapse by seeking support from someone who will help you avoid drinking while helping you deal with the loss you have suffered.

When my mother passed, I did not heed this advice and ended up overdrinking from the second I woke up the morning of the funeral. I did not speak at her funeral, which I regret to this day.

Environmental Triggers

- Bar / Club
- Friends' house
- BBQ
- Family Reunions
- The Lake

Environmental triggers are places that cause you to crave alcohol. A bar or nightclub is one of the most common addiction-triggering environments for many of us. This is because bars and nightclubs are structured to encourage the consumption of alcohol. To resist cravings, you either need to avoid going to these areas or devise a plan to help you resist the urge to drink while you're there. Aside from identifying your triggers, you will also need to prepare for the different reactions to your newfound sobriety from those who have only known you as a drunk.

Trigger Plan

Trigger Identification

List the times when you are most tempted to drink. Here are a few examples:

"I am tempted to drink _____"

Check off the statements that best apply to your drinking habits.

- When I am bored
- When I grieve
- When I am mad
- After work (you have perfect attendance at happy hour)
- When I am worried about a life situation
- When I see alcohol or others drinking alcohol
- When on vacation
- When my friends are drinking

Next, number them in order of strength. **One (1)** being the most likely to cause you to drink; **Ten (10)** being the least influential.

1. After work (you have perfect attendance at happy hour)
2. When I am bored
3. When my friends are drinking
4. When I see others drinking alcohol
5. When on vacation
6. When I grieve
7. When I am worried about a life situation
8. When I am mad

The second I got off work, my mouth would start to water. Securing a drink for the ride home was mandatory. Even if I had alcohol at the house, I never drove straight home. I had to hit the liquor store immediately after work. It was always my first stop.

When I am angry, it's not to say that I wouldn't be drinking, but I was usually focused on whatever made me upset to be triggered to drink. This is why it is at #10 as the least influential on my drinking.

Next, list the people, places, and things that might trigger you to relapse

Relapse Triggers	
People	Best friend Sibling / relative Coworkers Fraternity brothers Sorors/ Girlfriends
Places	After hours spot Bar Club BBQ
Things	Thinking about a lost one Regret Completion of a challenging task

If unavoidable, what will you do to lessen the chances of relapse?

If you don't know what to do who can you contact that does?

Have you Googled a solution? Online research?

I wanted to give you a few ways to inventory and analyze the hate in your life. These exercises will help you better understand your relationship with alcohol and give you a plan that can lead you toward a consistent life of sobriety. Through self-discovery, we can take more dominion over our lives.

Step 4: CONNECT

"The power of community to create health is far greater than any physician, clinic or hospital."
— *Mark Hyman, M.D.*

That which is monitored is managed

Peter Drucker, one of history's most prolific authors on business management, once wrote, "That which is measured is managed." Although this quote was originally intended to apply to the business world, we can use this as a guide toward managing our sobriety. In Alcoholics Anonymous, everyone knows their "day" or the first day of sobriety and can tell you exactly how long they have been sober. This knowledge helps to serve as a motivating factor. It is the reason we keep score during sporting events; it is the reason we weigh ourselves when attempting to lose weight. This principle can help you stay aware and motivated to sustain your commitment to your sobriety. Below are a few ways you can monitor your sobriety.

1) Calendar Tracking

When I first worked to increase content creation for my social media pages, I decided to establish a goal: I wanted to be sure to post one form of original content every day. When I first started, I figured all I needed to do was be sure to post every day and I'd be good. I did ok for the first few days, but as soon as "something came up," as it always does when you are living life, my consistency was destroyed. I relapsed back to a place of zero productivity.

Upon analyzing my reason for the inconsistency, I realized that I needed to do something different to achieve sustainability. This is when I ran across Peter Ducker's quote while reading a business blog. I then decided to get back to posting once daily but added a new action to my agenda. I purchased a calendar and every day after I completed my post, I would mark an "X" on the calendar for that day.

This act served a few functions that were conducive to my consistency. First, it helped me manage my actions because I was able to count the string of days I had posted in a row. When looking at the calendar month I was more motivated to stay consistent because I didn't want to see any "holes" in my calendar. I went from focusing on completing a week of posts to a month. I wanted to see a complete month with every day marked off.

There were times flying back and forth to California to see my kids that I had to post on social media while I was at the airport to keep my streak alive. But I was motivated to do it.

2) Gamify your sobriety

When I started teaching middle school, most students disliked test days. You could see the anxiety on the kid's faces as they prepared for what they felt to be impending doom. Some kids would even act up in an attempt to get sent to the office and avoid having to take tests. One thing I did to help them with this anxiety was to give them a more empowered perspective on the test and learning in general.

Think about a video game. It starts with some sort of challenge and goal. The difficulty increases as you pass through levels until you meet "The Final Boss." This is no different from a test except that kids enjoy playing games, yet they loathe taking tests. I had football players in my class that loved going to practice to prepare for their games but hated homework. I had to find a way to get them to buy into their education. After a few years and some research, I decided to change the way I spoke about their classwork, homework, and tests. I figured out that a game and a test absolutely had no significant structural difference. They measure skill, are challenging, involve some understanding of rules and regulations, can increase in difficulty, and are available for replay upon failure. The significant difference is in how they are perceived.

I started referring to classwork as 'practice' (math practice instead of math work). I was their coach, teaching them how to run plays, good study habits, absorb information, and test-taking skills. Test day became Game day.

Video Game	Test
• Measures skill • Challenging • Involves rules and regulations • Can increase in difficulty • Available for replay upon failure • **PERCEIVED AS FUN**	• Measures skill • Challenging • Involves rules and regulations • Can increase in difficulty • Available for replay upon failure • **PERCEIVED AS A BURDEN**

For humans, games have a positive inference. Games infer fun, excitement, and challenge. If a game only had one easily beatable level, then after beating it a few times it would become boring. Tests in school are no different but unlike games, tests are perceived as burdensome. To empower my students' perspective on the tests I would gamify my tests and refer to them as such while also letting them know that if they don't do well at the "game" there would be opportunities to replay and improve. View the scoreboard on the next page:

First 48 (hours)	Day 1				Day 2			
Level 1: 7 Days	☐	☐	☐	☐	☐	☐	☐	
Level 2: 14 Days	☐	☐	☐	☐	☐	☐	☐	
Level 3: 30 Days ☐	☐	☐	☐	☐	☐	☐	☐	☐
	☐	☐	☐	☐	☐	☐	☐	☐
Level 4: 60 Days ☐	Target Date:	Signature:						
Level 5: 100 days ☐	Target Date:	Signature:						
Level 6: 120 Days ☐	Target Date:	Signature:						
Level 7: 160 Days ☐	Target Date:	Signature:						
Level 8: 200 Days ☐	Target Date:	Signature:						
Level 9: 300 Days ☐	Target Date:	Signature:						
Level 10: 365 Days ☐	Target Date:	Signature:						

As you can see, lengths of time have been separated into "levels" that you can work to get to throughout the year. Marking down each day gives you a small reward for achieving a certain level similar to marking an "X" on a calendar. Scoreboards have been proven to help keep players engaged by keeping them in tune with their progress.

3) Mobile applications

I Am Sober:

The *I Am Sober* app is a great way to track your sober days via mobile phone. It also comes with other features that help keep you motivated and can connect you to a community of other "Sober Soldiers" that are working on attaining and maintaining their sobriety as well. Through this app, you can learn from others and share insights, tactics, and strategies. Some of the features include a Sober day tracker, Daily Pledge tracker, Sobriety Calculator, a Milestone tracker, and an area where you can share your story with others. It comes in a free and fee-based version with added features. *I Am Sober* is available for iOS and Android phones.

Days – Sobriety Counter

Days is a very simple and easy personal sobriety counter application that allows you to see the length of your sobriety in days, weeks, months, and years, either individually or combined. If you have been sober for any length of time, *Days* gives you the option to override your counter by either providing a new number of days or a new start date. For those who don't need many extras outside of a simple tracker, *Days* is quick and clean.

Building Your Village

"The power of community is most accurately measured by the compassion of its members."

— *Coretta Scott King*

Sobriety as a team sport

Sports in general and team sports specifically hold a place of high regard in the Black community. Many Black youth grow up aspiring to make it to "The League" primarily the NFL (National Football League) or the NBA (National Basketball Association). These professional players are lionized and worshipped by not only other Brothers and Sisters but also people of all races and ethnicities worldwide. In low-income Black neighborhoods, aside from music, sports are seen as the best chance for children to "make it out." It has been said that the only time a Black male can fully express his manhood is in war and in the arena. Just as with building an NBA dynasty, it is often necessary to acquire certain players to play certain positions and get rid of certain players to have a cohesive unit capable of winning; building your sober support group is no different.

Cutting and Bulking in Sobriety

In fitness, one of the most effective ways to gain muscle mass and lose body fat is a technique called bulking and cutting. Many people have used "bulking" and "cutting" cycles to reach a more aesthetically pleasing physique.

During the bulking cycle, bodybuilders will increase their caloric intake by eating more than usual while engaging in heavy lifting. The extra food supplies the amount of protein and nutrients needed to make the muscles grow. Although bulking stimulates muscle growth it also involves an amount of unwanted fat gain, which is why it is then followed by a cutting cycle. As the name implies, the cutting cycle involves eating at a caloric deficit and adjusting your workouts to burn fat while keeping as much of your hard-earned muscle and strength as possible. The goal of the cutting cycle is to get lean and remove excess body fat. The process of bulking and cutting also occurs in sobriety, with a cutting season usually preceding a season of bulking.

Cutting Season

In early sobriety you are likely to experience a cutting season. First, old drinking buddies that share your alcohol addiction but have no intention of quitting will start to leave your life voluntarily. This is because the social glue of alcohol is no longer shared between you. These are the people that may use with you but won't MOVE with you. Their only true bond to you is your old addiction and once that's gone, they're gone.

Although this is great for your sobriety it can hurt as people close to you may become distant, or even try to undermine your sobriety. This can be hard but will ultimately benefit and become easier to deal with in time. Allow these people to leave, the loyal friends that are willing to accept and respect your sober choice will eventually return as many of my friends did. Their leaving gave me more room to strengthen my sobriety and for that I am grateful, you will be too.

In this season you need to actively cut off toxic individuals that may be enemies of your sobriety. Some of your old drinking buddies may not leave on their own so you may need to help them out the door. Here are a few types of individuals that you need to cut to strengthen your chances of sustained sobriety:

1. People that don't respect your sober choice such as:

- Those who joke about your sobriety
- Those that try to undermine your sobriety through social pressure
- Those that try to have you justify your sober choice repeatedly

2. Alcoholics that have no intention of quitting.
3. Pessimists - People with a negative view of life in general are contagious.
4. Dry drunks - People that are sober but perpetually miserable because they have not addressed the factors that brought them to drink and have yet to look for or find a suitable alternative coping strategy, so they suffer in sobriety. They speak about their drinking days to the point of reminiscing. Be mindful of the amount of time you spend with them. Dry drunks often end up relapsing and will drag you to relapse with them if you're not careful.

Think about the people you drank with the most and assess whether they reflect any of the traits listed above. Any uncomfortable truths you uncover could ultimately be the reason you become and stay sober. Remember, your sobriety comes first. As social creatures, having these people cut from your life can produce a void. You can feel lonely, depressed and frustrated. This can be addressed in your next season of recovery, the bulking season.

Bulking Season

In your bulking season you become more active in your recovery. You'll meet people that share your interest in and respect for your sobriety. You begin to make healthier friends, learning new things and setting up new norms for your life. You will begin to meet new people that only know you as a non-drinker. These people will encourage you to continue in sobriety. You will "bulk up" on refreshing connections with great people if you make the effort to do so while continuing to cut off people that are bad for you.

While it's great to associate with other recovering alcoholics, be mindful of how they deal with adversity in their lives and be especially careful about entering a romantic relationship with someone in recovery. If you are in a relationship with somebody in recovery that seems headed towards a relapse either encourage them to get help. If they won't seek help for themselves you should sever ties. Protect YOUR sobriety at all cost!

Defining your current relationships

Most people in your social circle are in it because they all share the same interests. As the saying goes: "Birds of a feather flock together," For an alcoholic, this means that most of your best buddies are drinking buddies.

Make a list of your friends starting with the ones you spend the most time with. Next, add on people you see every once in a while, all the way down to the associates you don't see often. Identify the ones that don't drink, or rarely drink. You may want to try to find a way to spend more time with these people and less time with those you drink with the most.

Many people who have struggled with attaining sobriety in the past have said that they don't know anybody in their social circle who doesn't drink. Identify people in your life who are not dependent on drinking to have a good time. This can be made evident in the fact that you rarely see them drinking but they still hang out at the same places and go to the same events as you. These people are the types of people that you can go out with and not worry about increased social pressure to drink because they're not pressured to drink. They will join you while you're out having a good time and can enjoy themselves without having to go to the bar every other minute.

I was fortunate enough to have a few good friends that understood my struggle and helped me remain social without the pressure of having to drink. Since they usually didn't drink as often as I do, I didn't feel like I was impeding their good time. In our community, being able to socialize without drinking is a significant obstacle and challenge in our fight for sobriety. Alcohol has permeated our community through television advertisements, music, and celebrity-endorsed ads. It has been associated with money, success, sex, and power. Building a circle of friends willing to help you in your struggle and walk that road with you will help make your sobriety journey more manageable.

One person I consider a brother who doesn't drink regularly is Bert. In college, Bert attended all the same events as me, enjoying the same nights without having to worry about being hung over the next morning because he rarely drinks. He didn't need to and, therefore, never pressured me to drink when we were hanging out together. Once he knew I was fighting for sobriety, he was 100% supportive. For this reason, I was able to trust him, confide in him and get support when I felt the urge to drink. I understand that many are not as lucky. Having friends like Bert helped build my empowered perspective on sobriety.

It is good to have a support system of other people that are struggling so that you have a common goal. It is also important to find people that are living the version of healthy life you wish to achieve so that you can also set goals. Bishop T.D. Jakes talks about three types of relationships: confidantes, comrades, and constituents.

Constituents are people you associate with that share the same likes as you. For instance, two Laker fans would be constituents while they're at a Laker game. They may high-five each other every time their team scores a bucket, but once in the parking lot going back to their individual lives that relationship is over. If the person from the game saw you stranded on the side of the road with your Laker jersey on needing help with a flat tire, he may pull over and help you because you guys were both fans rooting for the same team at the game. If you were at the same game with the opposing team's jersey and rooting for them, the same constituent that aligned himself with you at the previous game would view you as more of an enemy, and the chances of him stopping to help you stranded on the side of the road with a Celtics jersey on are next to impossible. (As it should be... Go Lakers!)

Comrades share the same enemies as you. Soldiers in the same platoon are comrades on the battlefield. They are both there to defeat a common enemy. After the war is over and everyone returns to civilian life, the relationship ceases to exist. Your comrades are with you as long as you share the same enemy. Two members of the same gang usually surround themselves with a common enemy. Their friendship is centered on the fact that you have a common enemy you were both trying to defeat.

Confidantes are people whom you can confide in. They are with you and for you and give you advice from the heart. They may not share your same tastes in music, sports teams, food, clothes, or even religious beliefs, but they care about you and will always tell you what's best for you even if they know you don't want to hear it. Most parents fall in this category. Confidants are few and far between. If you have more than five you are blessed, and if you have none, you are in the majority.

Some of my drinking buddies were my constituents because we were bound together by alcohol consumption--both enemies of sobriety. Once I decided to no longer drink alcohol, our relationship started to weaken because we no longer had alcohol consumption in common. We lost our reason for hanging around one another. It is also why I initially faced resistance to my sobriety from friends and family. My drinking buddies would suggest moderation instead of sobriety. Some outright laughed at me and said that I would never be able to stick with it.

One of the fundamental mistakes people often make is to treat constituents like confidants. We tell these people our deepest secrets and it bonds us together but doesn't benefit us because the truth we often need to hear would only come from true confidants. What connected me to my constituents was alcohol. I never anticipated that my relationships with certain people would dwindle once I chose to stop drinking. After a few relapses and a greater understanding of how to delineate between constituents, comrades, and confidants, I was able to deal with their presence and absence from my life.

Your Sober Social Support Group

Psychological Safety

Google is not only a search engine but also a company known for conducting extensive analysis of their employees and the factors that contribute to a solid and collaborative working environment. They have looked at everything from the top-performing managers' shared characteristics to how often particular people within the company eat together. The company's initial goal was to uncover the most efficient way to construct the "Perfect team."

In 2012, Google created Project Aristotle, a year-long study that included interviews with hundreds of employees to analyze data about more than 100 active teams within the company.

According to Abeer Dubey, the manager of Google's People Analytics division at the time, Google looked at 180 teams from all over the company, but they found no evidence of a particular mix of specific personality types, skills, or backgrounds that made any difference. The 'who' part of the equation didn't seem to matter; what they did find was that "in the best teams, members show sensitivity, and most importantly, listen to one another."

A midlevel manager at Google, Matt Sakaguchi, decided to put Project Aristotle's findings into practice. He took his team off-site to open up about his cancer diagnosis. After a moment of hesitance, his colleagues then began sharing their own cancer stories.

Sakaguchi's strategy pointed to a concept known as "psychological safety," a shared belief that the team is safe for interpersonal risk-taking. Google found psychological safety to be a major contributing factor in building successful teams. For Google, building successful teams has less to do with who is in a team and more with how the members interact.

Conversely, to build your sobriety support network, you will need to find people that offer you the psychological safety of understanding the importance of your goal and who are willing to support that goal actively. Just as a sports team have different positions that are responsible for covering various aspects of the game. This support can come in many forms based on need and situation. I will now identify the roles or positions you may look to fill when building your sobriety support network.

1. Sober Soldiers (Comrades – enemy = Drinking Alcohol)

Sober soldiers are your brothers and sisters in arms who, like you, are fighting the same fight. They, too, have suffered from alcohol abuse and are working to live a life of sobriety. These are the people at the *Alcoholics Anonymous* meetings sitting next to you or in your virtual group who genuinely desire to quit drinking. They are your friends who can relate to your struggle because they are also going through it. Through mutual support, you can help one another do the work needed to attain and stay sober. You can go out with them knowing that they, too, have no intention to tempt you to relapse as they are working to avoid relapse. They are the comrades in the trenches with you fighting the same enemy—alcohol use and relapse.

Bill W. had been sober a few months when he began having strong cravings that were leading him to the verge of relapse. He felt, however, that if he could help another alcoholic, it would help him stay sober too. The endeavor of one drunk helping another was so successful that it led to the growth of one of the largest community-based self-help movements, *Alcoholics Anonymous*. 86 years of success has shown the power of enlisting the help of sober soldiers in this war for sobriety. Joining an AA group, finding peers that are also in recovery and helping them are great ways to immediately build your army of mutual sobriety support. They are your first line of defense

2. **Elders (sponsor) Confidants**

Elders are those who have been living a life of sobriety for many years and have a track record for maintaining their sobriety. These are the bridge builders that have experienced, endured, and overcome many of the challenges that one will face over years of sobriety. They have usually not only been sober for an extended amount of time but have also been to therapy to thoroughly address the underlying issues that caused them to abuse alcohol. An Elder will reason with you. An elder is someone you respect and hold in high regard who will give you advice and guidance from a place of genuine concern, void of any personal ulterior motives or agendas. You respect their opinion so you listen and consider whatever advice or guidance they may have for you. They are sober soldiers with years under their belts and a track record for helping others. They are also parental figures willing to take the time to help you renew your mind when it reaches out for an empowering perspective. **They are your confidants.**

The following poem explains the character of a true Elder:

The Bridge Builder

By William Allen Dromgoole

An old man going a lone highway,

Came, at the evening cold and gray,

To a chasm vast and deep and wide.

Through which was flowing a sullen tide

The old man crossed in the twilight dim,

The sullen stream had no fear for him;

But he turned when safe on the other side

And built a bridge to span the tide.

"Old man," said a fellow pilgrim near,

"You are wasting your strength with building here;

Your journey will end with the ending day,

You never again will pass this way;

You've crossed the chasm, deep and wide,

Why build this bridge at evening tide?"

The builder lifted his old gray head;

"Good friend, in the path I have come," he said,

"There followed after me to-day

A youth whose feet must pass this way.

This chasm that has been as naught to me

To that fair-haired youth may a pitfall be;

He, too, must cross in the twilight dim;

Good friend, I am building this bridge for him!"

3. **Neutral / Conductors (neutral environments)**

Neutrals are people you may not have a close relationship with but are important nonetheless because they create environments when drinking is not made a priority. You can find neutrals in environments where drinking alcohol is not allowed or socially accepted, such as a church, organized sporting events where you are participating (not a spectator), workshops, or volunteer groups.

Neutrals are found in low triggering environments. They are gathered in places where drinking would be seen as out of place. There is usually some purpose that has brought neutrals together that conflict with addictions. A greater purpose lies at the center of environments where you will find neutrals. This will help you keep your focus on the present purpose and not your addiction. Workout partners at fitness gyms, intermural sports teams, volunteer groups, social justice organizations, and even gun clubs are groups full of neutrals to provide a form of positive peer pressure by way of purpose and design.

4. **Enforcers**

These are people who are willing to physically stop you from taking a drink if you attempt to backslide in their presence. If you constantly get in the way of your own sobriety, I suggest you find and make an agreement with an enforcer while sober. They are a great "last line of defense" for those times when you actively attempt to backslide. Enforcers are usually necessary in the worst cases and must be people that you love. There are chemical enforcers such as prescription medicine Antabuse that causes sickness for anyone on it attempting to drink alcohol. (You must talk to your doctor to see if a prescription for Antabuse is necessary.) Enforcers are an option **only** for the worst cases of alcoholism where death is a relevant risk.

I started thinking about alternative ways to celebrate my wins and deal with my losses. One major way to deal with losses is to shift your focus to the solution. A great way to distract yourself from your addiction is to have a team of people you can bounce ideas off of to solve whatever he's got you in a negative mood. You **must** distract yourself from your addiction. When celebrating, think about other things you do to reward yourself and if you don't have anything this is a great time to start developing new rewards to replace your old reward of drinking.

Self-improvement is a great addiction to replace your old one. I jumped headfirst into self-improvement because it gave me purpose. Purpose is the key to living a sober life. When you have a purpose, you have other things for your mind to focus on and your body to be prepared for that will distract you from your addiction. Initially, I did not know where to start but knew I wanted to improve.

Step 5: KEEP

We got turned down, we failed, had setbacks, had to start over a lot of times, But we kept going at it. In anybody's case, that's always the distinguishing factor.
– Nipsey Hussle

KEEP ON,

KEEP AT IT,

AND IF YOU RELAPSE

KEEP COMING BACK

– SOBRIETY IN BLACK –

The Relapses

The first time I relapsed was on New Year's Eve, 2008. I had survived the Thanksgiving and Christmas holidays and was two months sober when an older friend of mine pulled up to the New Year's party I was attending (with all of my "former" drinking buddies), got out of the car, and immediately handed me a gallon jug of orange juice mixed with vodka. He was already drunk and simply said, "drink!". Without a second thought, I immediately decided to take a drink. I could have resisted, but in my mind, I found what I saw as a perfect excuse. The next morning, I awakened ashamed of my fall from grace due to my lack of discipline. I quickly got over that shame with the help of some leftover E&J and coke from the night before and continued with my life of drinking. The next year, I received my second DUI (center median mashup) and then made and failed my second attempt at sobriety.

When I relapsed the first time, I was very disappointed in myself. As I had stated earlier, 70% of those attempting sobriety will relapse in the first year. Most, if not all, who make the transition to an alcohol-free life, including myself, will relapse at some point. Relapse is a part of the recovery process. The beauty in the game of sobriety is that if you are among the living, you are always granted an opportunity to try again, to renew your commitment to sobriety. It took me three attempts before I could reach my current ten-year streak, so do not feel discouraged if you relapse. If you relapse, the best thing to do is to take inventory of the trigger(s): what caused you to drink. Then, put together a plan of action in case the challenge presents itself again in the future.

Sobriety is Never Owned

In 2004, after getting married, my wife and I purchased a modest single-family home in San Bernardino, California. One year later, I gained a new neighbor whom we'll call "Johnny" for the purposes of this book. After serving ten years, Johnny had recently been released from prison and was making a new life for himself, just as I had started my new life as a married man. Johnny and I talked daily about everything from his life in prison to his current situation dealing with family and his old gang. I would tell him about my life as a newlywed and my experiences in my fraternity, which he had asked about after seeing my frat brothers come by often for educational sessions with new prospects and step show practices.

Once when I offered him a beer, Johnny declined to explain that he stayed sober for his entire ten-year prison stint and had no intentions of picking up drinking again. He talked about how he could have engaged in drinking "Pruno" (prison wine made from fermented fruit) but chose not to because he couldn't afford to be intoxicated in there. He said he saw way too many people end up dead or victimized because of conflicts that arose while drinking, so he left it alone.

Unfortunately, within six months of living next to us as a free man, I noticed he had started drinking. His well-manicured lawn and clear driveway gave way to stray beer cans. Although I was drinking at the time, I then chose *never* to drink with him. We were always cordial, but something told me that this was a habit I *did not* want to start between us.

Over the next couple of months, his demeanor changed quickly. The seemingly stable guy I had first met had become much more unstable in his life, and the noise that once came primarily from my home started to come from his. One day I came home and noticed he was no longer around. My guess was that he was rearrested and sent back to prison for a violation because I saw police cars outside his house a few days after his disappearance. I now believe God sent him to give me a bird's-eye view of my potential future had I not turned my life around.

I once read a meme on Instagram that stated, "Sobriety is never owned; it's rented, and rent is due every day." In the comment section, a reader had noted her disdain for the meme, feeling it wasn't empowering, as if sobriety was temporary and not really ours. I, too, had a similar unease at the thought that sobriety was not mine to own.

This statement seemed to lack power and confidence, yet I felt as if there was a point I might be missing. So, I sat with it, pondering the point of the quote. I asked myself, "What could be the 'rent' due to maintaining my sobriety?" What would I need to 'pay' every day to maintain sobriety?

Then it hit me: *Mindfulness* is the price one must pay to maintain sobriety.

Mindfulness is the quality or state of being conscious or aware of something. Johnny had gone a long time without drinking and forgot he still had a drinking problem. During his ten years in prison, his motivation to cease drinking was not centered on his being mindful that he had a drinking problem but on the predators that could take advantage of him in prison while intoxicated. With that threat removed, his reason to stop drinking was no longer relevant in his mind.

Those recovering from alcohol addiction must remember that one drink will most likely lead to overdrinking. Being mindful of this every day is crucial to making a permanent improvement that comes with sobriety. To not fall "off the wagon," you cannot forget that you must *stay* on the wagon. You must be mindful that the wagon exists and that, for you, there can be dire consequences for drinking. A lack of constant mindfulness is why people can be sober for years only to return to drinking.

Famous actor Robin Williams talked about how he fell into a drinking binge after 20 years of sobriety. He wasn't mindful of the fact that drinking was not for him. He was rich and famous but forgot that money and fame could not buy sobriety, just as they cannot buy happiness. These things must be created by the individual and, like a garden or lawn, must be watered with mindfulness and self-awareness that keeps one on track. As the saying goes, "Never forget where you come from." This includes the losses you suffered in your war with alcohol. Once you start to live alcohol-free, you can never forget this fact: The consequences of drinking never disappear because you stop.

When working toward a life of consistent sobriety, you want to remember that this is a lifelong endeavor. There will not be a day when you "achieve" sobriety. There's no final level in this game as it is ongoing. The victory is in staying on the path of sobriety. Sobriety is a state of mind, not a fixed state of being. You must be mindful to work at it consistently to remain a winner. If you relapse, you can choose to walk in the right direction and reclaim your victory. Just like when driving somewhere, if you find out you are going in the wrong direction, you can always change your direction and end up on the correct path.

Renew, Review, Refocus and Reclaim

A relapse can be difficult to deal with. You will have feelings of inadequacy and may experience guilt brought on by the disappointment some may feel towards you after seeing you sober for a time and witnessing your relapse. Doubt will try to make its way into your mind and have you asking yourself, "Is it worth it?" Will I ever be able to shake this alcohol dependence?" You must understand that relapse is part of recovery as withdrawal and discomfort. The key is not to let it cause you to give up but use it as a learning experience. The positive thing about a relapse is that you now have identified an area you can work on to improve your chances of sustained sobriety. You can't fix an issue you never knew existed. This relapse brings information to you about an area for improvement that you may not have known before. You need to renew your commitment to sobriety, review your areas of concern, refocus your energy and actions on a corrective path, and regain your sobriety! Unlike a video game, you have another chance to reach new levels of sobriety every day!

Renew

In the previous section, I discussed the 12 Superpowers of sobriety. The twelfth Superpower, the Power of Renewal, is the most precious of all the superpowers because it's the one that you never lose. It never leaves you. Once you decide to take the road to sobriety, no matter how many times you fail, you never lose the Superpower of renewal.

Through renewal, you have a valuable opportunity to learn what triggered your relapse, what happens if the trigger comes again, and what will you do differently. Will you ask other people to help you? If you haven't tried it before, you could consider joining an AA group. Maybe find and establish a sponsor or talk to a relative, supportive friend, or confidant; these people want to see you win. Sobriety is a day-to-day process, so every second you're not drinking or succumbing to your addiction is a win. The power of renewal helps you learn from the past and appreciate the present so that you can have a greater future. You can do that by renewing your commitment to sobriety, reviewing your areas of concern, refocusing your energy on corrective actions, and regaining your sobriety.

Renewing your commitment simply means telling yourself, "I'm going to learn from my mistakes and try again." Renew your commitment to yourself first. If you are not doing it first for yourself, you are more likely to relapse. Understanding your value and appreciating yourself is essential. Without this, you will find no value in your love for others. If you feel worthless, what value can your love have to others? The same can be said about the value of your sobriety. If you do not see a personally redemptive value in your sobriety, you will eventually lose it and may fall back into the trap of alcohol dependency. Your sobriety must matter to you so it can be sustained.

- Renew your commitment to yourself to continue to fight for your sobriety
- Renew your commitment to your children to stay sober
- Renew your commitment to your loved ones (spouse, mother, friends) and understand why your sobriety will help you and others.

Review

Reviewing the situation that triggered your relapse is important because you want to avoid repeating your mistakes. Regardless of the situation, psychological, social, or emotional factors likely contributed to your craving to drink. You want to be honest enough with yourself to identify and assess all of the factors that lead to your relapse so that you can come up with an appropriate plan of action for the future. Use the experience as a learning moment to get the most out of it. Below is a list of questions you want to answer to get a better idea of what exactly lead you to relapse.

- Describe the event where you decided to take a drink
- What was going on?
- Describe the environment
- Were you by yourself or with other people? Where are they drinking?
- Describe your emotional state at the time of relapse. Where you:
- Happy?
- Sad?

- Anxious?
- Nervous?
- Grieving?
- Bored?
- Depressed?

Drinking is often the symptom of underlying problems in your life. For alcoholics and those that overindulge, it becomes a coping mechanism. Drinking helps us escape our negative feelings, numb pain associated with life, relax, or deal with anxiety, fears, and frustrations. To maintain sobriety, it is important to replace your current coping mechanism of drinking with other safe mechanisms. One way to do this is to find new ways to occupy your time and expend energy. Many people take on boxing, working out, or sports for aggression. For mental issues, some use journaling to express themselves. Consider alternative actions to prevent yourself from drinking.

Refocus (The Power of Purpose)

Focusing on your purpose is a great way to battle addiction. When you have purpose, you have focus; when you have focus, you are usually more easily distracted from your addiction. I realize that when I started focusing on my business, working out, improving my health, and coping skills, my mind stayed off alcohol. It was only when I lost sight of my purpose that I found myself craving alcohol.

In the Black community, survival is our primary purpose. Where other groups are often more secure in their survival, for us, it can be a full-time job. We are prone to moving more than any other demographic thanks to gentrification and redlining, are often discriminated against at our jobs, and are often prone to less stable living situations compared to other demographics. This can leave us with little time to search for purpose outside of tending to our basic needs, but it is essential to achieving true peace of mind, especially when fighting addiction.

To find your purpose, you will need to do some self-discovery. This can be rewarding because it allows you to try things you have never done before while contributing to your basic needs directly and indirectly. If what you do every day does not give you a sense of purpose, then it is time for you to look at other things to do or new events, new environments, new types of people, new activities, or hobbies that may help bring out your purpose.

The time you spent engaging in your addiction needs to be replaced with constructive activity. Consider possible hobbies that would help divert your attention from drinking:

1. An activity that makes money – I got into making and selling ammo
2. An activity that to keep you in shape – an exercise regimen
3. A creativity-based activity – Make music, write poetry
4. An activity that builds knowledge – Study my ancestral heritage
5. An activity that strengthens your mindset is meditation, self–control, discipline, etc.
6. A team / Family based activity – Escape rooms, meet-ups, etc.

List of activities

Hobbies to make money
    Start an online business
    Investing in stocks or crypto
    Sell items on social media platforms (Instagram shops, Facebook Marketplace)
    Start a consultancy firm based on your area of employment
    Start a blog

        Benefits: Increased financial independence, increased confidence, financial security

Hobbies to keep you in shape
    Gym Membership
    Hiking
    Walking
    Mountain bike riding

        Benefits: Improved health, increased confidence,

Hobbies to keep you creative
    Expressive writing (Journaling, poetry, etc.)
    Painting class
    Cook dishes from cookbooks from different countries
    Create your own "mocktails" (Non-alcoholic cocktails)

Benefits – Improved mental health, improved learning, and memorization, immune system boost

Hobbies to build knowledge
Reading
Watching documentaries (Complete "10 things I learned about…" worksheet)
Learn a new language

Benefits: Increased confidence, potential to find new opportunities, increased life satisfaction

Hobbies to strengthen your mindset
Meditation
Online courses centered on mental health
Study the Psychology of Happiness
Volunteering to help others in need
Benefits: Decreased stress, increased confidence
Social / Group-centered Hobbies
Intermural sports (Bowling League)
Online Gaming
Meetups
Book Club
Benefits: Strengthen social skills without alcohol

In the boxes below, think about six hobbies you could pursue based on the examples:

Types of Hobbies	Your Hobbies
Hobby to make money Hobby to keep you in shape Hobby to keep you creative Hobby to build knowledge Hobby to strengthen your mindset Hobbies to strengthen your social life	

Reclaim

Remember, you weren't born an alcoholic, and therefore, we are all working to reclaim the same sobriety we were born with. Even if you started drinking at age 12, for the first 11 years of your life, you lived, had fun, and faced adversity in your life without the need for alcohol. This means that you are simply relearning something you had at one time known before. Keep that in mind whenever you question the possibility of you living an alcohol-free life.

With your relapse review, trigger plan, and list of purpose-based activities, you will be in a strong position to finally retire from your career as an alcoholic. It's time to reclaim the sobriety you deserve not only for yourself but for the friends and family that love you as well!

You weren't *born* an alcoholic; you *became* an alcoholic. Now, it's time to get back to being your true self. There *is* Hope!

Medicinal Options

Disclaimer

In the interest of full disclosure, I need to make a statement regarding this particular section.

My editor, Georgina, whose work and opinion I highly respect, had suggested that since I am not a medical doctor, I should refrain from presenting the information in this chapter. At first, I was going to take her advice but then decided against it for the very reason I wrote it to begin with. The fact is, no medical professionals are explaining to the people or even informing the public about these medicinal options. So, I feel I must.

While methadone and other forms of medicines are prescribed to drug addicts, I find it unfortunate that there is little to no mention of these aforementioned medicines for those who suffer from alcoholism. These medicines could help some of the people suffering from the most severe cases of alcoholism where only a pharmaceutical intervention would be suitable and effective. I believe that all alcoholics should have an idea of the whole gamut of options that lie at their disposal. These medicines are not illegal but are available via prescription. Without knowledge of these options, one wouldn't even know to ask if they are available. I believe that this lack of knowledge is by design and on purpose. I would be more than happy to converse with medical professionals, legal professionals, and whoever is involved in the decision to suppress this information.

Society has no problem allowing us to drink, drive, live, and die as alcoholics but does not offer us the solutions that could be most effective for extreme cases. Author Neely Fuller Jr. defines justice as "making sure that no one is harmed at any time in any way and ensuring that those that need the most help get the most help." I believe that knowledge of these options is the best way to ensure that those who need the most help can get the most benefit. In all fairness to my editor, I wanted to make that clear so that any legal or social ramifications as to the printing of this particular section of the book sit whole-heartedly on my shoulders. Although she suggested I not put it in the book, I decided to do so on my own. I plan on spreading more information about these medicinal options to inform the public of all the options at our disposal as alcoholics.

"You don't have commercials talking about [these drugs]," says Stephen Holt, MD, co-director of the Addiction Recovery Clinic at Yale-New Haven Hospital St. Raphael Campus in Connecticut. "And primary care doctors tend to shy away from these meds because they weren't trained to use them in med school."

According to the CDC:

"Excessive alcohol use is responsible for more than 95,000 deaths in the United States yearly, or 261 deaths per day. These deaths shorten the lives of those who die by an average of almost 29 years, for a total of 2.8 million years of potential life lost. It is a leading cause of preventable death in the United States.

It is interesting to note that while you are inundated daily with commercials for medicines of all kinds, with all types of side effects, you have never seen commercials for medicines that could help cure dependence on a substance that is the leading cause of preventable deaths in the United States.

Disulfiram

According to WedMD.com, Disulfiram was the first drug that the FDA approved for alcohol use disorder. Disulfiram is the active ingredient in prescription drugs commonly known as Antabuse. It changes the way your body breaks down alcohol. If you drink while taking it, you get sick. Whole Antabuse is effective in bringing pleasure out of drinking; it is also this discomfort that makes it hard to stick to.

Naltrexone

According to the US Department of Health and Human Services Substance Abuse and Mental Health Services Administration (SAMHSA), Naltrexone is an FDA-approved medication prescribed to treat both alcohol use disorder (AUD) and opioid use disorder (OUD). It works by blocking the euphoric and sedative (read: "feel good") effects of opioids such as heroin, morphine, and codeine. This reduces cravings for drugs and alcohol.

With Naltrexone, you will still feel drunk if you drink, but you won't feel the pleasure that comes with being drunk. According to Holt, "Naltrexone can help uncouple alcohol and pleasure." Naltrexone can be taken daily as a pill or monthly by injection at your health care professional's office.

Naltrexone works best after you have been alcohol-free for at least four days to avoid strong side effects such as nausea and vomiting.

Acamprosate (Campral)

Acamprosate is used to ease withdrawal symptoms and stifle cravings during the initial stages of sobriety. It works by resetting the alcohol-induced imbalance between two chemical messenger systems in the brain: GABA (short for gamma-aminobutyric acid) and glutamate. To be effective, patients must take two pills three times a day.

Two other medications that are FDA approved to treat seizures but have been prescribed "off label" for alcohol use disorders are gabapentin and topiramate. Like acamprosate interact with GABA and glutamate systems. Studies show that they may help people avoid drinking, drink less, and have fewer cravings.

Recovering Loudly

When we recover loudly we help keep others from dying quietly -Unknown

Writing this book about my struggle with alcoholism and transformation in recovery has become a purpose that continues to reinforce my sobriety. It gives me the power to live without my addiction. This is why I believe everyone in recovery should write at least one book, a blog, social media post, or a video series to tell stories about the struggles they have experienced. This is a quick and straightforward way to turn the experiences that you have had, good or bad, into lessons to help someone else learn from your mistakes. The best way to learn a new task is to study it, then use the knowledge, and teach it to someone else.

A lighthouse on the open seas provides direction for lost ships looking for signs of land or life. Those lost at sea are given a viable choice of an effective direction to travel. As a lighthouse of sobriety, your examples, experience, and willingness to help others offer the same security. Friends and loved ones who may be suffering from the throws of addiction should be able to come to you for guidance or encouragement. You serve as an example of someone that continues to strive towards a goal they may wish to achieve. This may mean the difference between success and failure for those that know you. I was somewhat surprised at the number of people from my drinking past who would ask me how I could stay sober, endure relapse, and still maintain a fulfilling life in sobriety. Like a lighthouse, you can serve as a point of direction for someone who may not know exactly how to pursue sobriety.

It is my hope that this book can serve as a lighthouse to support those on their journey to sobriety.

And so, lifting as we climb, onward and upward we go, struggling and striving, and hoping that the buds and blossoms of our desires will burst into glorious fruition 'ere long. With courage, born of success achieved in the past, with a keen sense of responsibility, which we shall continue to assume, we look forward to a future large with promise and hope. - Mary Church Terrell

References

Beauvais F. (1998). American Indians and alcohol. *Alcohol health and research world*, *22*(4), 253–259.

Carmona, M. (Ed.). (2021, June 2). *Alcohol relapse rates: Abstinence statistics, how to avoid & deal with a relapse*. The Recovery Village Drug and Alcohol Rehab.

Centers for Disease Control and Prevention. (2020, October 1). *Deaths and years of potential life lost from excessive alcohol use - United States, 2011–2015*. Centers for Disease Control and Prevention.

Center on Alcohol Marketing and Youth. Youth Exposure to Alcohol Advertising in National Magazines, 2001-2008. Baltimore, MD; 2010.

Clear, J. (2018). *Atomic habits: An easy & proven way to build good habits & break bad ones*. Avery Publishing Group.

Collins, S. (2021, May 3). *Alcoholism medications and how they work*. WebMD.

Correa, G. (2021, March 24). *Addiction and Low-Income Americans*. Addiction Center.

Dingle, G. A., Cruwys, T., & Frings, D. (1AD, January 1). *Social identities as pathways into and out of addiction*. Frontiers.

Drake J, Charles C, Bourgeois JW, Daniel ES, Kwende M. Exploring the impact of the opioid epidemic in Black and Hispanic communities in the United States. Drug Science, Policy, and Law. January 2020. doi:10.1177/2050324520940428

Giles, C. (2021, May 28). *Opioids like 'lean' permeate hip-hop culture, but dangers are downplayed*. Kaiser Health News.

Scoro.com (2017, June 20). 7 Stories That Prove The Importance of Teamwork: After years of intensive analysis, Google discovers the key to good teamwork

Lacy, M. (1992, December 15). *Marketing of malt liquor fuels debate: Consumption: Sales of the high-alcohol beverage soar in inner cities. critics complain that shrewd advertising in ethnic neighborhoods has turned it into a status symbol.* Los Angeles Times.

Naltrexone. SAMHSA. (n.d.). https://www.samhsa.gov/medication-assisted-treatment/medications-counseling-related-conditions/naltrexone.

DuBois, W.E.B. (1896). *The Suppression of the African slave trade.* New York: Schocken. Greene, L. J. (1942). *The Negro in colonial New England.* New York: Columbia University

Press.

Duhigg, C. (2014). *The Power of Habit: Why we do what we do in life and business.* Random House Trade Paperbacks.

Junewicz, N. (2019, November 27). *FBI: Average drunk driver has driven drunk more than 80 times before first arrest.* WZTV. Retrieved November 3, 2021, from https://fox17.com/news/local/fbi-average-drunk-driver-has-driven-drunk-more-than-80-times-before-first-arrest.

Prochaska, J.O., Redding, C.A., & Evers, K. (2002). The Transtheoretical Model and Stages of Change. In K. Glanz, B.K. Rimer & F.M. Lewis, (Eds.) Health Behavior and Health Education: Theory, Research, and Practice (3rd Ed.). San Francisco, CA: Jossey-Bass, Inc.

Smith, K. C., Cukier, S., & Jernigan, D. H. (2014). Regulating alcohol advertising: Content analysis of the adequacy of federal and self-regulation of magazine advertiscments, 2008-2010. *American Journal of Public Health, 104*(10), 1901-11.

Wood-Wright, N., & JH Bloomberg School of Public Health. (2015, June 23). *African-American youth are exposed to more alcohol advertising than youth in general.* Johns Hopkins Bloomberg School of Public Health

Appendix

The following are direct excerpts from articles cited in this book. Although they were paraphrased in the book, I felt adding the excerpts may give some context to the information and decrease the chance of anything being "lost in translation."

INVOLVEMENT OF ALCOHOL DURING ENSLAVEMENT

Source: Christmon, K. (1995). Historical Overview of Alcohol in the African American Community. *Journal of Black Studies*, 25(3), 318–330. http://www.jstor.org/stable/2784640

In the United States, slavery is usually associated with the southern region. The rigorous climate in New England, the character of the settlers, and their political views served to discourage the use of Africans as slaves. New England's role in slavery lies not in its use of Africans as enslaved people but in the fact that New Englanders were the traders in enslaved Africans for the new world. Crucial to the "slave trade" and New England's economy were rum and molasses. Rum was New England's largest manufacturing business before the Revolutionary War (Greene, 1942). New England furnished enslaved Africans to the other colonies (DuBois, 1896). Rhode Island and Massachusetts had more than 22 and 63 stills, and these two states became the leading importers of Africans and the leading exporters of rum (DuBois, 1896). In 1770, New England exports of rum to Africa represented more than four-fifths of the total colonial export of the year (Williams, 1944). Rum, which is distilled from molasses, was an essential part of the cargo of the slave ship, particularly American slave ships. No slave trader could afford to leave the New England dock without a cargo of rum aboard the ship (Greene, 1942). The rum trade on the coast became a virtual monopoly for New England.

Owners of slavers carried Africans to South Carolina and brought them back to New England naval stores for their shipbuilding or to the West Indies and brought back molasses. The molasses was made into the highly prized New England rum and shipped in hogsheads to Africa for more human cargo (DuBois, 1896, pp. 28-29). Thus, the American involvement is often referred to as the triangular slave trade. Twenty gallons of rum could purchase a muscular young man (Larkin, 1965). It was profitable to spread a taste for liquor on the coast. The African dealers, supplied with rum, were induced to drink until they lost their reason; then, the bargain was struck. One African dealer, his bag full of the gold paid to him for the capture of Africans, accepted the captain's invitation to dinner. He was made drunk and awoke the next morning to find his money gone, and himself stripped, branded, and enslaved with his victims, to the great mirth of the sailors (Williams, 1944).

As can be seen, alcohol was intricately tied to the "slave trade." Alcohol was used to the benefit of enslavers—to aid them in the captivity of Africans and, consequently, New England prospered.

USE OF ALCOHOL AND OTHER DRUGS DURING THE SLAVERY AND POSTSLAVERY ERAS IN THE UNITED STATES

Initially, Africans in the United States used alcohol and beer in religious ceremonies and rituals as practiced in Africa (Stuckey, 1987). However, as the number of Africans increased, European Americans began passing legislation restricting the use of alcohol by Africans. Restrictions applied to enslaved Africans and free Africans. By the middle of the 18th century, colonists had enacted measures to prevent Africans from drinking. In New Jersey, colonial statutes forbade Whites from selling or trading in rum with Blacks. Any person convicted of selling or giving rum or any strong liquor to African Americans became liable to a penalty of five pounds by law in 1692 (Williams, 1970). Such measures were based on the notion that Blacks were too irresponsible to be trusted with the use of alcohol and also on the fear that Blacks would be less accepting of the conditions of their servitude, more difficult to control, and prone to violence when inebriated.

After the American War of Independence, slavery was prohibited or nearly abolished in nearly all colonial governments, and consequently, more freedom with respect to alcohol ensued. However, by the beginning of the Civil War, slave-holding states prohibited or controlled the consumption of alcoholic beverages by Blacks (Brown & Tooley, 1989). The danger of mass drunkenness and the potential revolt was heightened following Nat Turner's and Denmark Vessey's revolts (Larkin, 1965). Laws were enacted that placed tighter controls on drinking and even prevented African Americans from owning stills. For example, South Carolina in 1831 passed a law prohibiting any free Black from owning or operating a still. This prohibition became unenforceable during the Civil War. Still, following the Civil War, African Americans were again prevented from owning alcoholic beverages in the southern states, although they had been granted the rights of citizenship.

Although European Americans tightly controlled the use of alcoholic beverages among Africans, enslaved and free, Africans were allowed to drink freely during holidays. Holidays, especially Christmas, were when the greatest amount of drinking was done by enslaved Africans (Johnson, 1937). Enslaved Africans would dance and drink until many of them passed out from drinking. Stroyer (1898, p. 45) wrote that both masters and the enslaved regarded Christmas as a great day. Africans typically received from five to six days off. There would be two or three large pails filled with sweetened water, with a gallon or two of whiskey in each; this was distributed to them until they were partly drunk.

In his autobiography, Frederick Douglass (1892) described that the days between Christmas and New Year's Day were allowed as holidays for enslaved Africans. During this time, owners made bets that an enslaved African could drink more whiskey than any other. They encouraged enslaved Africans to get drunk, and they discouraged them from doing anything that might be viewed as constructive. Large numbers of enslaved Africans drank until they passed out. Douglass adds that owners used alcohol to subdue and tranquilize enslaved Africans. In this way, Whites hoped to combat any movement toward insurrection. The use of alcohol accompanied by drunkenness was considered normal on those occasions.

Whites had contradictory attitudes toward alcohol and Africans. On the one hand, they believed that alcohol increased the Africans' propensity toward insurrection, for example, Nat Turner must have been under the influence of alcohol. On the other hand, slave owners believed that, by keeping the Africans intoxicated, especially during their free time, enslaved Africans would not have the opportunity to think about their plight and plan a rebellion. To some extent, owners managed to reconcile the two contradicting positions. European Americans controlled the production and distribution of alcohol among free and enslaved Africans. On holidays, enslaved Africans were able to drink, and slave owners would encourage drunkenness. Whites believed drunkenness would prevent Africans from thinking about their plight or doing anything that might lead to freedom. Owners were able to provide a certain amount of surveillance during these times. The use of alcohol during other times was extremely limited, and the penalty for drunken behavior was severe and often harsh.

After the Civil War ended in 1865, drinking and drunkenness were features in the lifestyle of the newly freed Africans. Profuse drinking and public drunkenness were not uncommon in the ranks of the formerly enslaved, but most African Americans practiced moderation (Koren, 1899). The drinking of alcoholic beverages in any amount by Blacks was generally resented in most communities. It was believed that liquor gave Blacks a false sense of being equal or superior to Whites, which was intolerable in the South (Larkin, 1965). Thus, Blacks exhibited comparatively low rates of alcohol use, drunkenness, and problems due to drinking. In this regard, chronic drunkenness was so rare among Blacks that they were thought physiologically immune from prolonged inebriety (Koren, 1899).

At the time of the temperance movement of the 19th century, African Americans had the lowest mortality rate due to alcoholism of any ethnic group. African Americans during this era tended to support temperance because the temperance movement stood against slavery (Larkin, 1965). In 1858, John Rock addressed a crowd: "The Negro who hangs around the corners of the streets or lives in the grog-shops . . . is forging fetters for the slave and is a curse to his race" (Rock, 1988). The platform of the temperance movement shifted from the northern abolitionists to poor rural southerners. Prohibitionists urged protecting Whites, particularly White women, from the drunken debauches of half-crazed men. Blacks detached themselves from the temperance movement and headed north to avoid the violence (Herd, 1983). Thus, at the turn of the century, when African Americans migrated from the South to the North, occasions for alcohol consumption were similar to that of pre-colonial Africa. Alcohol consumption among African Americans was low when compared to other groups, and drunken behavior was rare. African Americans used alcohol for ceremonial celebrations.

Blacks migrated in mass from the South to the North to escape from Jim Crowism and economic and political exploitation. However, African Americans encountered hostility and discrimination. The North turned out not to be the "promised land." They were crammed into inadequate living quarters and unable to find work. Also, taverns, as social outlets, began to take on greater significance in northern African-American communities than in the South. The patterns of alcohol use among African Americans began to shift. Since the late 1950s, there has been a rapid annual increase in the frequency of liver cirrhosis as a cause of death in Blacks (Herd, 1985). Cirrhosis of the liver is not always caused by excessive use of alcohol, yet it does provide a crude measure of alcoholism. Between 1950 and 1973, liver cirrhosis among Caucasians increased by 60%, and the rate among African Americans rose by 242% (Herd, 1985). Since 1973, the liver cirrhosis rates have leveled off, yet the rate among African Americans is still disproportionately high (Herd, 1986).

The Suppression of the African Slave Trade to The United States of America 1638–1870
Chapter IV: THE TRADING COLONIES.
New England and the Slave-Trade.

Vessels from Massachusetts,[1] Rhode Island,[2] Connecticut,[3] and, to a less extent, from New Hampshire,[4] were early and primarily engaged in the carrying slave trade.

"We know," said Thomas Pemberton in 1795, "that a large trade to Guinea was carried on for many years by the citizens of Massachusetts Colony, who were the proprietors of the vessels and their cargoes, out and home. Some of the enslaved people purchased in Guinea, and I suppose the greatest part of them, were sold in the West Indies."5 Dr. John Eliot asserted that "it made a considerable branch of our commerce. It declined very little till the Revolution."6 Yet the trade of this colony was said not to equal that of Rhode Island. Newport was the mart for enslaved people offered for sale in the North and a point of reshipment for all enslaved people. Principally, this trade raised Newport to its commercial importance in the eighteenth century.7 Connecticut, too, was a vital slave trader, sending large numbers of horses and other commodities to the West Indies in exchange for enslaved people and selling the enslaved people in other colonies.

This trade formed a perfect circle. Owners of slavers carried enslaved people to South Carolina and brought home naval stores for their shipbuilding, or to the West Indies and brought home molasses, or to other colonies and brought hogsheads. The molasses was made into the highly prized

New England rum and shipped in these hogsheads to Africa for more enslaved people.8 Thus, the rum-distilling industry indicates, to some extent, the activity of New England in the slave trade. In May 1752, one Captain Freeman found so many slavers fitting out that, despite the large importations of molasses, he could get no rum for his vessel.9 In Newport alone, twenty-two stills were at one time running continuously;10 and Massachusetts annually distilled 15,000 hogsheads of molasses into this "chief manufacture."11

The First Decade Of 'European Beer' In Apartheid South Africa: The State, The Brewers, And The Drinking Public, 1962–72

Abstract

The study of liquor provides an opportunity for re-examining relations between states and economies. Recent works in European social history have shown that liquor occupies an ambiguous space between economic, social, and cultural production. In contrast, studies of liquor in colonial Africa repeatedly raise the problem of how economic freedoms pertaining to liquor were constructed about the perceived character of persons in society. More specifically, the notion of 'European liquor' in colonial discourse suggests that the liquor of colonial masters should be aspired to. 'European liquor' was repeatedly contrasted to indigenous brews of lower alcoholic content, pronounced uncivilized and primitive. It implied that drinkers of sorghum beer, palm wine, and other beverages fermented from African grains and fruits would progress to the 'superior' beverages of their colonial masters. Critically, it assumed that transition to the higher alcoholic content required the discipline of 'European' lifestyles. Gradualism, however, often gave way to expediency. Colonial regimes repeatedly set aside fears of the effect of 'foreign' liquor on African subjects in the interest of revenue and political gains. The importation of gin by the colonial authority in Ghana provided the regime with revenue for its administration; in colonial Nigeria and elsewhere, liquor was used by the state to win allies among chiefs.

Made in the USA
Columbia, SC
25 June 2025